Children's Interview for Psychiatric Syndromes

Report Forms

PARENT VERSION

P-ChIPS

Also available from American Psychiatric Publishing Group (1-800-368-5777; www.appi.org)

■ **ChIPS—Children's Interview for Psychiatric Syndromes** (Order #8398)
(reusable interview administration booklet)

Based on strict DSM-IV criteria and validated in more than 12 years of studies, the ChIPS is brief and simple to administer. Questions are succinct, simply worded, and easily understood by children and adolescents. Practitioners in clinical and research settings alike have already found the ChIPS indispensable in screening for conditions such as attention-deficit/hyperactivity disorder, conduct disorder, substance abuse, phobias, anxiety disorders, stress disorders, eating disorders, mood disorders, elimination disorders, and schizophrenia.

Scoring Form for ChIPS, package of 20 (Order #8846)
(one-time-use booklet for recording answers, with Profile Sheet)

Scoring Forms provide ample space for recording verbatim responses to interview questions, with check boxes to indicate whether symptom criteria and duration and impairment requirements are met. A Profile Sheet, perforated for easy removal from the Scoring Form, is included to itemize principal findings and diagnoses.

Report Form for ChIPS, package of 20 (Order #8899)
(one-time-use abbreviated summary form)

Report Forms provide a quick way of conveying ChIPS results. If subsequently desired, this "at-a-glance" summary of the symptoms endorsed during the interview can be used by a clinician to identify areas warranting further scrutiny.

■ **P-ChIPS—Children's Interview for Psychiatric Syndromes—Parent Version** (Order #8847)
(reusable interview administration booklet)

The Parent Version of the ChIPS essentially consists of the same interview text altered from second to third person to address the parent rather than the child (e.g., "Have you ever" is changed to "Has your child ever").

Scoring Form for P-ChIPS, package of 20 (Order #8396)
(one-time-use booklet for recording answers, with Profile Sheet)

Report Form for P-ChIPS, package of 20 (Order #8399)
(one-time-use abbreviated summary form)

■ **Administration Manual** (Order #8849)

Covering both the ChIPS and the P-ChIPS, the Administration Manual is informative and user-friendly. It presents background information about the interview's development, detailed instructions for conducting the interview and recording its results, explicit criteria for assessing interviewee responses, complete specifications for preparing mental health paraprofessionals to administer the interview, and illustrative case studies.

ISBN 0-88048-399-7

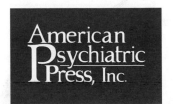

American Psychiatric Press, Inc.

ORDER/REORDER FORM

Order No.	Quantity	Title	Price	Total
8398	_____	**ChIPS - Children's Interview for Psychiatric Syndromes** (reusable interview administration booklet)	$39.95	$_____
8846	_____	**Scoring Form for ChIPS, package of 20** (one-time-use booklet for recording answers, with Profile Sheet)	$24.95	$_____
8899	_____	**Report Form for ChIPS, package of 20** (one-time-use abbreviated summary form)	$19.95	$_____
8847	_____	**P-ChIPS - Children's Interview for Psychiatric Syndromes — Parent Version** (reusable interview administration booklet)	$39.95	$_____
8396	_____	**Scoring Form for P-ChIPS, package of 20** (one-time-use booklet for recording answers, with Profile Sheet)	$24.95	$_____
8399	_____	**Report Form for P-ChIPS, package of 20** (one-time-use abbreviated summary form)	$19.95	$_____
8849	_____	**Administration Manual**	$24.95	$_____
8908	_____	**Starter Kit** (Includes ChIPS - Children's Interview for Psychiatric Syndromes; Scoring Form for ChIPS (package of 5); Report Form for P-ChIPS (package of 5); P-ChIPS - Children's Interview for Psychiatric Syndromes — Parent Version; Scoring Form for P-ChIPS (package of 5); and Report Form for P-ChIPS (package of 5)	$115.00	$_____

SHIPPING AND HANDLING

$25.00 or less......add $5.95	$75.00–$99.99......add $10.95
$25.01–$49.99....add $6.95	$100.00–$149.99..add $12.95
$50.00–$74.99....add $8.95	Over $150.00........add $15.95

All prices in U.S. Dollars. Orders must be prepaid and include shipping & handling. Allow 10 days for delivery. Contact Customer Service at 1-800-368-5777 for additional delivery options.

SUBTOTAL $_____

Tax* $_____

Plus Shipping and Handling $_____

TOTAL $_____

*Calculate tax on books:
District of Columbia residents add 5.75% tax;
Canadian residents add 7% GST.
In Canada: Please order through Login Bros. Canada, 324 Saulteaux Crescent, Winnipeg, Manitoba B3J 3T2
Phone Toll-Free: 1-800-665-1148 (24 hours a day)
Internet: http://www.lb.com
E-Mail: sales@lb.com

Please check method of payment

☐ Check Enclosed (Payable to *American Psychiatric Press, Inc.*)

Charge My ☐ Visa ☐ Mastercard ☐ American Express

Account #_____ Exp. Date _____/_____

Signature _____ Date _____

Send To: ☐ Business address ☐ Residential address
(Unless otherwise specified, all orders are shipped via UPS to street address—no P.O. boxes please.)

Name _____

Address _____

City _____

State/Province _____ Zip/Postal Code _____

Country _____

Phone _____ E-mail _____

☐ Please send me the 1999 American Psychiatric Publishing Group Catalog

☐ Please send me information on publications via e-mail

TO ORDER:

Cite title or set, order no., quantity and payment method (Visa, MC and AMEX accepted), add shipping and handling (per chart), and send your order via:

 MAIL: Complete the order form and mail it to us.

 PHONE: Call toll free at 1-800-368-5777, 9 am - 5 pm ET, Mon. - Fri.

 FAX: 202-789-2648, 24 hours a day.

 E-MAIL: order@appi.org

 INTERNET: Visit our World Wide Web site at http://www.appi.org and place your orders online.

Visit your local medical bookstore.

AMERICAN PSYCHIATRIC PUBLISHING GROUP
1400 K Street, NW
Washington, DC 20005

MDXB

P-ChIPS Report Form

Child's Name: _____ Date: _____ / _____ / _____

Informant's Name: _____ Interviewer: _____

Informant's Relationship (circle one): Mother, Father, Stepmother, Stepfather, Guardian, Other _____

Attention-Deficit/Hyperactivity Disorder

A: Inattention

1. a. pays no attention to details
   b. makes careless mistakes on schoolwork
2. can't keep mind on what he/she is doing
3. a. has trouble listening to parent
   b. has trouble listening to teacher
4. has trouble finishing things
5. has trouble organizing self
6. avoids schoolwork
7. loses school supplies
8. a. is easily distracted
   b. teacher reports inattention/daydreaming
9. a. is forgetful
   b. teacher reports forgetfulness

B: Hyperactivity–Impulsivity

1. a. is often told to sit still
   b. is constantly moving hands/feet
2. a. has trouble staying in seat
   b. gets in trouble for getting out of chair
3. gets in trouble for running/climbing
4. a. is too loud when playing
   b. has difficulty playing quietly
5. teacher reports is always "on the go"
6. a. talks out of turn at school
   b. talks too much at home
7. blurts out answers to questions
8. a. pushes ahead in line
   b. can't wait for his/her turn in games
9. a. barges in on other kids' games
   b. pushes into others' groups
   c. interrupts busy people

Oppositional Defiant Disorder

1. a. loses temper when things don't go his/her way
   b. has frequent temper tantrums
2. a. talks back/argues with parents
   b. talks back/argues with teachers
3. a. breaks rules at home
   b. breaks rules at school
   c. refuses to follow teachers' directions
   d. disobeys direct orders
4. purposely "bugs" other people
5. blames others for his/her own mistakes
6. is easily angered by others
7. is angry a lot of the time
8. gets even when angered

Conduct Disorder

1. has stolen >1 time
2. a. lies to get out of doing things
   b. "cons" people
3. has broken into a car or building to steal
4. has skipped school >3 times
5. breaks curfew >1 time per month
6. has run away/stayed out all night >1 time *or* did not return for a long time
7. a. is a bully
   b. threatens other people
8. a. is avoided because he/she starts fights
   b. gets in trouble for fighting
9. has used a weapon in a fight >1 time
10. a. has hurt someone badly in a fight
    b. has hurt someone for no reason
11. has taken things from people by force
12. has damaged property
13. has set something on fire (>1 time *or* caused extensive damage)
14. has hurt or killed an animal for fun
15. a. has forcefully performed sexual activity on another
    b. has forced someone to perform sexual activity on him-/herself

Substance Abuse

1. a. has smoked cigarettes ≥2 times _____
   b. has smoked pot ≥2 times _____
   c. has smoked other drugs ≥2 times _____
2. has used alcohol _____
3. has used other drugs _____
4. has sniffed a substance ≥2 times _____

Specific Phobia

1. phobic object/situation: _____
2. when confronted with object/situation,
   a. gets uptight and scared, can't move
   b. cries, clings to parents, throws tantrums
3. a. avoids object/situation
   b. becomes nauseated, feels faint
4. a. fear interferes with (sleep, school, activities)
   b. feels *super* uncomfortable because of fear
5. a. is more scared of object/situation than peers
   b. fear seems silly to child

Social Phobia

1. a. is afraid of being around other people
   b. has fear of performing
2. feels super-uncomfortable when a/b occurs
3. a. tries to avoid social situations
   b. if unavoidable, feels awful
4. a. fear interferes with (sleep, school, activities)
   b. feels *super* uncomfortable because of fear
5. behavior seems silly to child

Separation Anxiety

1. a. cries, begs parent to stay home
   b. tries to stay home with parent at all times
2. a. worries about parent getting harmed
   b. fears parental harm if separated
3. fears personal harm when separated from parent
4. a. has difficulty going to school
   b. refuses to go to school
5. a. is afraid to be in room of house alone
   b. follows parent around the house
6. a. can't sleep if not with parent
   b. can't sleep away from home
7. a. has nightmares about separation
   b. has nightmares about parental loss
8. a. has stomach- or headaches before going to school
   b. gets ill when parent leaves him/her

Generalized Anxiety Disorder

1. worries more than other kids _____
2. a. has difficulty calming down
   b. can't let go of worry
3. when worried, feels edgy, tired, distractible, cranky; has tight muscles, poor sleep

Obsessive-Compulsive Disorder

A: Compulsions

1. does things over and over
2. a. feels behavior will improve things
   b. thinks that if he/she can't perform behavior, something bad will happen
3. feels that behavior does not make sense

B: Obsessions

1. a. has bothersome thoughts/ideas
   b. "sees" pictures in head repeatedly
   c. has to do something but never does it
2. a. tries to make bothersome thoughts go away
   b. tries to pretend that thoughts aren't there
   c. does other things to try to make thoughts go away

3. thoughts seem like child's own (as opposed to someone else putting thoughts in his/her mind)

C: Interference

1. a. thoughts/behaviors cause child discomfort
   b. thoughts/behaviors cause problems at (home, school, play)
   c. thoughts/behaviors interfere with daily routines (time spent daily: _____)

Stress Disorders—PTSD, ASD

A: Exposure

1. a. child experienced traumatic event _____
   b. child witnessed traumatic event happening to someone else _____
2. after event, felt helpless, shocked, horrified, like he/she was falling apart; was hard to calm down
3. how long ago did event happen? _____

B: Dissociation

1. after event, felt cut off from family/friends; felt fewer emotions, felt numb
2. felt out of touch, in a daze
3. felt that the world was not real
4. felt that self was no longer real
5. had trouble remembering event

C: Reexperiencing

1. a. replays event over and over in mind
   b. "sees" event happening again
   c. plays games about event over and over
2. a. has nightmares about event
   b. has nightmares but can't remember what they're about
3. a. "feels" event happening again
   b. acts like event is happening again
4. a. becomes upset when reminded of event
   b. becomes upset when in same physical setting in which event occurred
5. when reminded of event, gets anxious, achy, sweaty palms, breathing problems

D: Avoidance

1. a. avoids thinking/talking about event
   b. tries to be unafraid of anything
2. a. avoids activities that remind him/her of event
   b. avoids places that remind him/her of event
   c. avoids people that remind him/her of event
3. can't remember things about event
4. a. has decreased interest in things he/she used to enjoy
   b. has stopped doing things he/she used to enjoy
5. feels cut off from family/friends
6. feels fewer emotions; feels numb
7. a. feels he/she won't grow up
   b. feels he/she will die soon

E: Hyperarousal

1. a. has trouble falling asleep
   b. has trouble staying asleep
2. a. is harder to get along with
   b. is easily angered
3. has difficulty concentrating
4. is super-alert
5. is easily startled, jumpy

Anorexia

1. a. has lost weight by dieting
   b. tries to stay underweight
2. a. current weight and height _____
   b. weight and height when thinnest _____
3. a. is terrified of getting fat
   b. is afraid of gaining weight
   c. fears he/she won't stop eating if he/she starts
4. a. feels fat
   b. feels good/bad depending on weight
   c. thinks his/her weight is a problem
5. if she's started menstruation yet, amenorrhea?

Bulimia

1. eats lots of food in short time
2. feels he/she can't stop eating, only stops because

   _____
3. after eating, tries to lose weight by . . .
   a. not eating
   b. vomiting
   c. taking laxatives
   d. overexercising
4. a. is more weight-conscious than peers
   b. self-image depends on weight

Depression/Dysthymia

A: Dysphoric Mood

1. a. feels sad or depressed
   b. almost every day
   c. lasts most of the day
2. a. feels more irritable
   b. (i) fights (ii) cries (iii) temper
   c. almost every day
   d. lasts most of the day

B: Loss of Interest

1. a. used to have fun doing _____
   b. isn't fun anymore
2. a. wants to have fun but can't
   b. feels that nothing is fun anymore
   c. has lost interest in daily activities

C: Appetite Changes

1. a. has decreased appetite
   b. has lost weight without dieting
   c. clothes are too big now
2. a. has increased appetite
   b. has gained weight

D: Sleep Changes

1. goes to bed @ _____; wakes @ _____
   a. early insomnia
   b. middle insomnia
   c. late insomnia
2. a. naps a lot
   b. hypersomnia

E: Psychomotor Changes

1. a. can't sit still
   b. is fidgety
   c. wrings hands
   d. picks at him-/herself
2. a. takes longer to do things
   b. has difficulty doing anything

F: Low Energy

1. a. has no energy
   b. has to push self
   c. tires easily
   d. sits around, does nothing

G: Guilt

1. a. has bad thoughts about self
   b. feels down on self
   c. feels he/she is no good
   d. hates self
2. a. feels guilty a lot
   b. thinks he/she should be punished

H: Impaired Concentration

1. a. mind has slowed down
   b. forgets things more
   c. has trouble paying attention
   d. listens to teacher less than before
   e. grades have dropped
2. has difficulty making up mind

I: Hopelessness

1. a. feels that nothing good will happen in the future
   b. feels that things won't get any better
   c. feels that there's no hope for the future

J: Morbid/Suicidal Thoughts

1. a. thinks about death
   b. thinks about dead people/pets
2. a. wishes he/she were dead
   b. feels life isn't worth living
   c. has thought of suicide
   d. has thought of suicide plans
   e. has made suicide attempt

Mania/Hypomania

A: Elevated Mood

1. a. feels very, very good
   b. feels wonderful for no reason
   c. is "too high"
2. has discrete periods of irritability

B: Other Symptoms

1. a. believes he/she has special abilities
   b. believes he/she can do things better than anyone
2. a. has lots of energy, no need for sleep
   b. sleeps a lot less without feeling tired
   c. needs ≤3 hours of sleep to feel OK
3. a. has rapid, unstoppable speech
   b. talks so fast that family/friends worry
   c. is told he/she talks too much, too loudly
   d. talks too fast to be understood
4. a. thoughts race through mind
   b. thoughts come too fast to verbalize them all
   c. feels that mind is sped up, working too fast
5. has trouble focusing
6. a. does more things than usual
   b. has more energy than usual
   c. tries many different things
   d. family/friends are concerned
   e. is more active than usual
7. a. gets in trouble more
   b. does things he/she usually wouldn't
   c. gets hurt due to carelessness
   d. is a lot more interested in sex than usual

C: Interference

1. mood/behavior causes problems at (home, school, play)
2. mood/behavior is reason child is here

Enuresis

1. has wet bed after kindergarten
2. a. wets bed at night
   b. wets self during day
3. a. occurs when not sick
   b. is not due to effects of some medication

Encopresis

1. has had bowel movement outside of toilet after kindergarten
2. happens when not sick

Schizophrenia/Psychosis

A: Psychotic Symptoms

1. a. feels someone is out to harm him/her
   b. feels someone is trying to make him/her sick
   c. people seem to be against him/her
   d. people seem to talk about him/her
   e. people spy on him/her
2. a. eyes play tricks on him/her
   b. during daylight
   c. only when falling asleep
   d. ears play tricks on him/her
   e. voices talk about child's feelings/thoughts/acts
   f. voices talk to each other

Interviewer observed:

3. *incoherent speech*
4. *disorganized or catatonic behavior*
5. *inappropriate affect or inability to speak*

B: Interference

1. since problems started, has more difficulty getting along with other people
2. since problems started, does worse in school
3. since problems started, is careless about looks/ hygiene

Psychosocial Stressors

A: Child Abuse/Neglect

1. a. M/F criticizes child a lot
   b. M/F wishes child had never been born
   c. M/F says he/she hates child
2. a. M/F ignores child
   b. M/F misses child's doctor appointments
   c. M/F does not feed child
   d. M/F does not clothe child
3. a. child is spanked or hit
   b. child is sometimes spanked or hit for no reason
   c. child fears physical harm from M/F
   d. child has been bruised, sore, taken to doctor
4. child has been sexually abused
5. child has been made to go a whole day without food

B: Other Stressors

1. a. fighting within family
   b. among children
   c. between parents
   d. between parents and children
   e. fighting bothers child
2. child remembers parents' separation/divorce
3. a. family has money problems
   b. child is worried about money problems
4. a. family member is ill
   b. family member has been hospitalized
   c. child worries
5. a. family member drinks or uses drugs a lot
   b. child worries
6. a. family member has been in trouble with police
   b. child worries
7. a. someone close to child has gotten sick and died
   b. child was very upset
8. a. someone close to child was murdered
   b. child was very upset
   c. someone close to child was killed in an accident
   d. child was very upset
9. anything else we need to know so we can help you?
   _____
   _____
10. problems child thinks he/she needs help with?
   _____
   _____
11. anything in the interview that bothered you?
   _____
   _____

P-ChIPS Report Form

Child's Name: _____ Date: ____ / _____ / _____

Informant's Name: _____ Interviewer: _____

Informant's Relationship (circle one): Mother, Father, Stepmother, Stepfather, Guardian, Other _____

Attention-Deficit/Hyperactivity Disorder

A: Inattention

1. a. pays no attention to details
   b. makes careless mistakes on schoolwork
2. can't keep mind on what he/she is doing
3. a. has trouble listening to parent
   b. has trouble listening to teacher
4. has trouble finishing things
5. has trouble organizing self
6. avoids schoolwork
7. loses school supplies
8. a. is easily distracted
   b. teacher reports inattention/daydreaming
9. a. is forgetful
   b. teacher reports forgetfulness

B: Hyperactivity–Impulsivity

1. a. is often told to sit still
   b. is constantly moving hands/feet
2. a. has trouble staying in seat
   b. gets in trouble for getting out of chair
3. gets in trouble for running/climbing
4. a. is too loud when playing
   b. has difficulty playing quietly
5. teacher reports is always "on the go"
6. a. talks out of turn at school
   b. talks too much at home
7. blurts out answers to questions
8. a. pushes ahead in line
   b. can't wait for his/her turn in games
9. a. barges in on other kids' games
   b. pushes into others' groups
   c. interrupts busy people

Oppositional Defiant Disorder

1. a. loses temper when things don't go his/her way
   b. has frequent temper tantrums
2. a. talks back/argues with parents
   b. talks back/argues with teachers
3. a. breaks rules at home
   b. breaks rules at school
   c. refuses to follow teachers' directions
   d. disobeys direct orders
4. purposely "bugs" other people
5. blames others for his/her own mistakes
6. is easily angered by others
7. is angry a lot of the time
8. gets even when angered

Conduct Disorder

1. has stolen >1 time
2. a. lies to get out of doing things
   b. "cons" people
3. has broken into a car or building to steal
4. has skipped school >3 times
5. breaks curfew >1 time per month
6. has run away/stayed out all night >1 time *or* did not return for a long time
7. a. is a bully
   b. threatens other people
8. a. is avoided because he/she starts fights
   b. gets in trouble for fighting
9. has used a weapon in a fight >1 time
10. a. has hurt someone badly in a fight
    b. has hurt someone for no reason
11. has taken things from people by force
12. has damaged property
13. has set something on fire (>1 time *or* caused extensive damage)
14. has hurt or killed an animal for fun
15. a. has forcefully performed sexual activity on another
    b. has forced someone to perform sexual activity on him-/herself

Substance Abuse

1. a. has smoked cigarettes ≥2 times _____
   b. has smoked pot ≥2 times _____
   c. has smoked other drugs ≥2 times _____
2. has used alcohol _____
3. has used other drugs _____
4. has sniffed a substance ≥2 times _____

Specific Phobia

1. phobic object/situation: _____
2. when confronted with object/situation,
   a. gets uptight and scared, can't move
   b. cries, clings to parents, throws tantrums
3. a. avoids object/situation
   b. becomes nauseated, feels faint
4. a. fear interferes with (sleep, school, activities)
   b. feels *super* uncomfortable because of fear
5. a. is more scared of object/situation than peers
   b. fear seems silly to child

Social Phobia

1. a. is afraid of being around other people
   b. has fear of performing
2. feels super-uncomfortable when a/b occurs
3. a. tries to avoid social situations
   b. if unavoidable, feels awful
4. a. fear interferes with (sleep, school, activities)
   b. feels *super* uncomfortable because of fear
5. behavior seems silly to child

Separation Anxiety

1. a. cries, begs parent to stay home
   b. tries to stay home with parent at all times
2. a. worries about parent getting harmed
   b. fears parental harm if separated
3. fears personal harm when separated from parent
4. a. has difficulty going to school
   b. refuses to go to school
5. a. is afraid to be in room of house alone
   b. follows parent around the house
6. a. can't sleep if not with parent
   b. can't sleep away from home
7. a. has nightmares about separation
   b. has nightmares about parental loss
8. a. has stomach- or headaches before going to school
   b. gets ill when parent leaves him/her

Generalized Anxiety Disorder

1. worries more than other kids _____
2. a. has difficulty calming down
   b. can't let go of worry
3. when worried, feels edgy, tired, distractible, cranky; has tight muscles, poor sleep

Obsessive-Compulsive Disorder

A: Compulsions

1. does things over and over
2. a. feels behavior will improve things
   b. thinks that if he/she can't perform behavior, something bad will happen
3. feels that behavior does not make sense

B: Obsessions

1. a. has bothersome thoughts/ideas
   b. "sees" pictures in head repeatedly
   c. has to do something but never does it
2. a. tries to make bothersome thoughts go away
   b. tries to pretend that thoughts aren't there
   c. does other things to try to make thoughts go away

3. thoughts seem like child's own (as opposed to someone else putting thoughts in his/her mind)

C: Interference

1. a. thoughts/behaviors cause child discomfort
   b. thoughts/behaviors cause problems at (home, school, play)
   c. thoughts/behaviors interfere with daily routines (time spent daily: _____)

Stress Disorders—PTSD, ASD

A: Exposure

1. a. child experienced traumatic event _____
   b. child witnessed traumatic event happening to someone else _____
2. after event, felt helpless, shocked, horrified, like he/she was falling apart; was hard to calm down
3. how long ago did event happen? _____

B: Dissociation

1. after event, felt cut off from family/friends; felt fewer emotions, felt numb
2. felt out of touch, in a daze
3. felt that the world was not real
4. felt that self was no longer real
5. had trouble remembering event

C: Reexperiencing

1. a. replays event over and over in mind
   b. "sees" event happening again
   c. plays games about event over and over
2. a. has nightmares about event
   b. has nightmares but can't remember what they're about
3. a. "feels" event happening again
   b. acts like event is happening again
4. a. becomes upset when reminded of event
   b. becomes upset when in same physical setting in which event occurred
5. when reminded of event, gets anxious, achy, sweaty palms, breathing problems

D: Avoidance

1. a. avoids thinking/talking about event
   b. tries to be unafraid of anything
2. a. avoids activities that remind him/her of event
   b. avoids places that remind him/her of event
   c. avoids people that remind him/her of event
3. can't remember things about event
4. a. has decreased interest in things he/she used to enjoy
   b. has stopped doing things he/she used to enjoy
5. feels cut off from family/friends
6. feels fewer emotions; feels numb
7. a. feels he/she won't grow up
   b. feels he/she will die soon

E: Hyperarousal

1. a. has trouble falling asleep
   b. has trouble staying asleep
2. a. is harder to get along with
   b. is easily angered
3. has difficulty concentrating
4. is super-alert
5. is easily startled, jumpy

Anorexia

1. a. has lost weight by dieting
   b. tries to stay underweight
2. a. current weight and height _____
   b. weight and height when thinnest _____
3. a. is terrified of getting fat
   b. is afraid of gaining weight
   c. fears he/she won't stop eating if he/she starts
4. a. feels fat
   b. feels good/bad depending on weight
   c. thinks his/her weight is a problem
5. if she's started menstruation yet, amenorrhea?

Bulimia

1. eats lots of food in short time
2. feels he/she can't stop eating, only stops because
   _____
3. after eating, tries to lose weight by . . .
   a. not eating
   b. vomiting
   c. taking laxatives
   d. overexercising
4. a. is more weight-conscious than peers
   b. self-image depends on weight

Depression/Dysthymia

A: Dysphoric Mood
1. a. feels sad or depressed
   b. almost every day
   c. lasts most of the day
2. a. feels more irritable
   b. (i) fights (ii) cries (iii) temper
   c. almost every day
   d. lasts most of the day

B: Loss of Interest
1. a. used to have fun doing _____
   b. isn't fun anymore
2. a. wants to have fun but can't
   b. feels that nothing is fun anymore
   c. has lost interest in daily activities

C: Appetite Changes
1. a. has decreased appetite
   b. has lost weight without dieting
   c. clothes are too big now
2. a. has increased appetite
   b. has gained weight

D: Sleep Changes
1. goes to bed @ _____; wakes @ _____
   a. early insomnia
   b. middle insomnia
   c. late insomnia
2. a. naps a lot
   b. hypersomnia

E: Psychomotor Changes
1. a. can't sit still
   b. is fidgety
   c. wrings hands
   d. picks at him-/herself
2. a. takes longer to do things
   b. has difficulty doing anything

F: Low Energy
1. a. has no energy
   b. has to push self
   c. tires easily
   d. sits around, does nothing

G: Guilt
1. a. has bad thoughts about self
   b. feels down on self
   c. feels he/she is no good
   d. hates self
2. a. feels guilty a lot
   b. thinks he/she should be punished

H: Impaired Concentration
1. a. mind has slowed down
   b. forgets things more
   c. has trouble paying attention
   d. listens to teacher less than before
   e. grades have dropped
2. has difficulty making up mind

I: Hopelessness
1. a. feels that nothing good will happen in the future
   b. feels that things won't get any better
   c. feels that there's no hope for the future

J: Morbid/Suicidal Thoughts
1. a. thinks about death
   b. thinks about dead people/pets
2. a. wishes he/she were dead
   b. feels life isn't worth living
   c. has thought of suicide
   d. has thought of suicide plans
   e. has made suicide attempt

Mania/Hypomania

A: Elevated Mood
1. a. feels very, very good
   b. feels wonderful for no reason
   c. is "too high"
2. has discrete periods of irritability

B: Other Symptoms
1. a. believes he/she has special abilities
   b. believes he/she can do things better than anyone
2. a. has lots of energy, no need for sleep
   b. sleeps a lot less without feeling tired
   c. needs ≤3 hours of sleep to feel OK
3. a. has rapid, unstoppable speech
   b. talks so fast that family/friends worry
   c. is told he/she talks too much, too loudly
   d. talks too fast to be understood
4. a. thoughts race through mind
   b. thoughts come too fast to verbalize them all
   c. feels that mind is sped up, working too fast
5. has trouble focusing
6. a. does more things than usual
   b. has more energy than usual
   c. tries many different things
   d. family/friends are concerned
   e. is more active than usual
7. a. gets in trouble more
   b. does things he/she usually wouldn't
   c. gets hurt due to carelessness
   d. is a lot more interested in sex than usual

C: Interference
1. mood/behavior causes problems at (home, school, play)
2. mood/behavior is reason child is here

Enuresis

1. has wet bed after kindergarten
2. a. wets bed at night
   b. wets self during day
3. a. occurs when not sick
   b. is not due to effects of some medication

Encopresis

1. has had bowel movement outside of toilet after kindergarten
2. happens when not sick

Schizophrenia/Psychosis

A: Psychotic Symptoms

1. a. feels someone is out to harm him/her
   b. feels someone is trying to make him/her sick
   c. people seem to be against him/her
   d. people seem to talk about him/her
   e. people spy on him/her
2. a. eyes play tricks on him/her
   b. during daylight
   c. only when falling asleep
   d. ears play tricks on him/her
   e. voices talk about child's feelings/thoughts/acts
   f. voices talk to each other

Interviewer observed:
3. *incoherent speech*
4. *disorganized or catatonic behavior*
5. *inappropriate affect or inability to speak*

B: Interference

1. since problems started, has more difficulty getting along with other people
2. since problems started, does worse in school
3. since problems started, is careless about looks/ hygiene

Psychosocial Stressors

A: Child Abuse/Neglect

1. a. M/F criticizes child a lot
   b. M/F wishes child had never been born
   c. M/F says he/she hates child
2. a. M/F ignores child
   b. M/F misses child's doctor appointments
   c. M/F does not feed child
   d. M/F does not clothe child
3. a. child is spanked or hit
   b. child is sometimes spanked or hit for no reason
   c. child fears physical harm from M/F
   d. child has been bruised, sore, taken to doctor
4. child has been sexually abused
5. child has been made to go a whole day without food

B: Other Stressors

1. a. fighting within family
   b. among children
   c. between parents
   d. between parents and children
   e. fighting bothers child
2. child remembers parents' separation/divorce
3. a. family has money problems
   b. child is worried about money problems
4. a. family member is ill
   b. family member has been hospitalized
   c. child worries
5. a. family member drinks or uses drugs a lot
   b. child worries
6. a. family member has been in trouble with police
   b. child worries
7. a. someone close to child has gotten sick and died
   b. child was very upset
8. a. someone close to child was murdered
   b. child was very upset
   c. someone close to child was killed in an accident
   d. child was very upset
9. anything else we need to know so we can help you?
   _____
   _____
10. problems child thinks he/she needs help with?
    _____
    _____
11. anything in the interview that bothered you?
    _____
    _____

P-ChIPS Report Form

Child's Name: _____ Date: ____ / _____ / _____

Informant's Name: _____ Interviewer: _____

Informant's Relationship (circle one): Mother, Father, Stepmother, Stepfather, Guardian, Other _____

Attention-Deficit/Hyperactivity Disorder

A: Inattention

1. a. pays no attention to details
   b. makes careless mistakes on schoolwork
2. can't keep mind on what he/she is doing
3. a. has trouble listening to parent
   b. has trouble listening to teacher
4. has trouble finishing things
5. has trouble organizing self
6. avoids schoolwork
7. loses school supplies
8. a. is easily distracted
   b. teacher reports inattention/daydreaming
9. a. is forgetful
   b. teacher reports forgetfulness

B: Hyperactivity–Impulsivity

1. a. is often told to sit still
   b. is constantly moving hands/feet
2. a. has trouble staying in seat
   b. gets in trouble for getting out of chair
3. gets in trouble for running/climbing
4. a. is too loud when playing
   b. has difficulty playing quietly
5. teacher reports is always "on the go"
6. a. talks out of turn at school
   b. talks too much at home
7. blurts out answers to questions
8. a. pushes ahead in line
   b. can't wait for his/her turn in games
9. a. barges in on other kids' games
   b. pushes into others' groups
   c. interrupts busy people

Oppositional Defiant Disorder

1. a. loses temper when things don't go his/her way
   b. has frequent temper tantrums
2. a. talks back/argues with parents
   b. talks back/argues with teachers
3. a. breaks rules at home
   b. breaks rules at school
   c. refuses to follow teachers' directions
   d. disobeys direct orders
4. purposely "bugs" other people
5. blames others for his/her own mistakes
6. is easily angered by others
7. is angry a lot of the time
8. gets even when angered

Conduct Disorder

1. has stolen >1 time
2. a. lies to get out of doing things
   b. "cons" people
3. has broken into a car or building to steal
4. has skipped school >3 times
5. breaks curfew >1 time per month
6. has run away/stayed out all night >1 time *or* did not return for a long time
7. a. is a bully
   b. threatens other people
8. a. is avoided because he/she starts fights
   b. gets in trouble for fighting
9. has used a weapon in a fight >1 time
10. a. has hurt someone badly in a fight
    b. has hurt someone for no reason
11. has taken things from people by force
12. has damaged property
13. has set something on fire (>1 time *or* caused extensive damage)
14. has hurt or killed an animal for fun
15. a. has forcefully performed sexual activity on another
    b. has forced someone to perform sexual activity on him-/herself

Substance Abuse

1. a. has smoked cigarettes ≥2 times _____
   b. has smoked pot ≥2 times _____
   c. has smoked other drugs ≥2 times _____
2. has used alcohol _____
3. has used other drugs _____
4. has sniffed a substance ≥2 times _____

Specific Phobia

1. phobic object/situation: _____
2. when confronted with object/situation,
   a. gets uptight and scared, can't move
   b. cries, clings to parents, throws tantrums
3. a. avoids object/situation
   b. becomes nauseated, feels faint
4. a. fear interferes with (sleep, school, activities)
   b. feels *super* uncomfortable because of fear
5. a. is more scared of object/situation than peers
   b. fear seems silly to child

Social Phobia

1. a. is afraid of being around other people
   b. has fear of performing
2. feels super-uncomfortable when a/b occurs
3. a. tries to avoid social situations
   b. if unavoidable, feels awful
4. a. fear interferes with (sleep, school, activities)
   b. feels *super* uncomfortable because of fear
5. behavior seems silly to child

Separation Anxiety

1. a. cries, begs parent to stay home
   b. tries to stay home with parent at all times
2. a. worries about parent getting harmed
   b. fears parental harm if separated
3. fears personal harm when separated from parent
4. a. has difficulty going to school
   b. refuses to go to school
5. a. is afraid to be in room of house alone
   b. follows parent around the house
6. a. can't sleep if not with parent
   b. can't sleep away from home
7. a. has nightmares about separation
   b. has nightmares about parental loss
8. a. has stomach- or headaches before going to school
   b. gets ill when parent leaves him/her

Generalized Anxiety Disorder

1. worries more than other kids _____
2. a. has difficulty calming down
   b. can't let go of worry
3. when worried, feels edgy, tired, distractible, cranky; has tight muscles, poor sleep

Obsessive-Compulsive Disorder

A: Compulsions

1. does things over and over
2. a. feels behavior will improve things
   b. thinks that if he/she can't perform behavior, something bad will happen
3. feels that behavior does not make sense

B: Obsessions

1. a. has bothersome thoughts/ideas
   b. "sees" pictures in head repeatedly
   c. has to do something but never does it
2. a. tries to make bothersome thoughts go away
   b. tries to pretend that thoughts aren't there
   c. does other things to try to make thoughts go away

3. thoughts seem like child's own (as opposed to someone else putting thoughts in his/her mind)

C: Interference

1. a. thoughts/behaviors cause child discomfort
   b. thoughts/behaviors cause problems at (home, school, play)
   c. thoughts/behaviors interfere with daily routines (time spent daily: _____)

Stress Disorders—PTSD, ASD

A: Exposure

1. a. child experienced traumatic event _____
   b. child witnessed traumatic event happening to someone else _____
2. after event, felt helpless, shocked, horrified, like he/she was falling apart; was hard to calm down
3. how long ago did event happen? _____

B: Dissociation

1. after event, felt cut off from family/friends; felt fewer emotions, felt numb
2. felt out of touch, in a daze
3. felt that the world was not real
4. felt that self was no longer real
5. had trouble remembering event

C: Reexperiencing

1. a. replays event over and over in mind
   b. "sees" event happening again
   c. plays games about event over and over
2. a. has nightmares about event
   b. has nightmares but can't remember what they're about
3. a. "feels" event happening again
   b. acts like event is happening again
4. a. becomes upset when reminded of event
   b. becomes upset when in same physical setting in which event occurred
5. when reminded of event, gets anxious, achy, sweaty palms, breathing problems

D: Avoidance

1. a. avoids thinking/talking about event
   b. tries to be unafraid of anything
2. a. avoids activities that remind him/her of event
   b. avoids places that remind him/her of event
   c. avoids people that remind him/her of event
3. can't remember things about event
4. a. has decreased interest in things he/she used to enjoy
   b. has stopped doing things he/she used to enjoy
5. feels cut off from family/friends
6. feels fewer emotions; feels numb
7. a. feels he/she won't grow up
   b. feels he/she will die soon

E: Hyperarousal

1. a. has trouble falling asleep
   b. has trouble staying asleep
2. a. is harder to get along with
   b. is easily angered
3. has difficulty concentrating
4. is super-alert
5. is easily startled, jumpy

P-ChIPS

Anorexia

1. a. has lost weight by dieting
   b. tries to stay underweight
2. a. current weight and height _____
   b. weight and height when thinnest _____
3. a. is terrified of getting fat
   b. is afraid of gaining weight
   c. fears he/she won't stop eating if he/she starts
4. a. feels fat
   b. feels good/bad depending on weight
   c. thinks his/her weight is a problem
5. if she's started menstruation yet, amenorrhea?

Bulimia

1. eats lots of food in short time
2. feels he/she can't stop eating, only stops because

   _____
3. after eating, tries to lose weight by . . .
   a. not eating
   b. vomiting
   c. taking laxatives
   d. overexercising
4. a. is more weight-conscious than peers
   b. self-image depends on weight

Depression/Dysthymia

A: Dysphoric Mood
1. a. feels sad or depressed
   b. almost every day
   c. lasts most of the day
2. a. feels more irritable
   b. (i) fights (ii) cries (iii) temper
   c. almost every day
   d. lasts most of the day

B: Loss of Interest
1. a. used to have fun doing _____
   b. isn't fun anymore
2. a. wants to have fun but can't
   b. feels that nothing is fun anymore
   c. has lost interest in daily activities

C: Appetite Changes
1. a. has decreased appetite
   b. has lost weight without dieting
   c. clothes are too big now
2. a. has increased appetite
   b. has gained weight

D: Sleep Changes
1. goes to bed @ _____; wakes @ _____
   a. early insomnia
   b. middle insomnia
   c. late insomnia
2. a. naps a lot
   b. hypersomnia

E: Psychomotor Changes
1. a. can't sit still
   b. is fidgety
   c. wrings hands
   d. picks at him-/herself
2. a. takes longer to do things
   b. has difficulty doing anything

F: Low Energy
1. a. has no energy
   b. has to push self
   c. tires easily
   d. sits around, does nothing

G: Guilt
1. a. has bad thoughts about self
   b. feels down on self
   c. feels he/she is no good
   d. hates self
2. a. feels guilty a lot
   b. thinks he/she should be punished

H: Impaired Concentration
1. a. mind has slowed down
   b. forgets things more
   c. has trouble paying attention
   d. listens to teacher less than before
   e. grades have dropped
2. has difficulty making up mind

I: Hopelessness
1. a. feels that nothing good will happen in the future
   b. feels that things won't get any better
   c. feels that there's no hope for the future

J: Morbid/Suicidal Thoughts
1. a. thinks about death
   b. thinks about dead people/pets
2. a. wishes he/she were dead
   b. feels life isn't worth living
   c. has thought of suicide
   d. has thought of suicide plans
   e. has made suicide attempt

Mania/Hypomania

A: Elevated Mood
1. a. feels very, very good
   b. feels wonderful for no reason
   c. is "too high"
2. has discrete periods of irritability

B: Other Symptoms
1. a. believes he/she has special abilities
   b. believes he/she can do things better than anyone
2. a. has lots of energy, no need for sleep
   b. sleeps a lot less without feeling tired
   c. needs ≤3 hours of sleep to feel OK
3. a. has rapid, unstoppable speech
   b. talks so fast that family/friends worry
   c. is told he/she talks too much, too loudly
   d. talks too fast to be understood
4. a. thoughts race through mind
   b. thoughts come too fast to verbalize them all
   c. feels that mind is sped up, working too fast
5. has trouble focusing
6. a. does more things than usual
   b. has more energy than usual
   c. tries many different things
   d. family/friends are concerned
   e. is more active than usual
7. a. gets in trouble more
   b. does things he/she usually wouldn't
   c. gets hurt due to carelessness
   d. is a lot more interested in sex than usual

C: Interference
1. mood/behavior causes problems at (home, school, play)
2. mood/behavior is reason child is here

Enuresis

1. has wet bed after kindergarten
2. a. wets bed at night
   b. wets self during day
3. a. occurs when not sick
   b. is not due to effects of some medication

Encopresis

1. has had bowel movement outside of toilet after kindergarten
2. happens when not sick

Schizophrenia/Psychosis

A: Psychotic Symptoms

1. a. feels someone is out to harm him/her
   b. feels someone is trying to make him/her sick
   c. people seem to be against him/her
   d. people seem to talk about him/her
   e. people spy on him/her
2. a. eyes play tricks on him/her
   b. during daylight
   c. only when falling asleep
   d. ears play tricks on him/her
   e. voices talk about child's feelings/thoughts/acts
   f. voices talk to each other

Interviewer observed:

3. *incoherent speech*
4. *disorganized or catatonic behavior*
5. *inappropriate affect or inability to speak*

B: Interference

1. since problems started, has more difficulty getting along with other people
2. since problems started, does worse in school
3. since problems started, is careless about looks/ hygiene

Psychosocial Stressors

A: Child Abuse/Neglect

1. a. M/F criticizes child a lot
   b. M/F wishes child had never been born
   c. M/F says he/she hates child
2. a. M/F ignores child
   b. M/F misses child's doctor appointments
   c. M/F does not feed child
   d. M/F does not clothe child
3. a. child is spanked or hit
   b. child is sometimes spanked or hit for no reason
   c. child fears physical harm from M/F
   d. child has been bruised, sore, taken to doctor
4. child has been sexually abused
5. child has been made to go a whole day without food

B: Other Stressors

1. a. fighting within family
   b. among children
   c. between parents
   d. between parents and children
   e. fighting bothers child
2. child remembers parents' separation/divorce
3. a. family has money problems
   b. child is worried about money problems
4. a. family member is ill
   b. family member has been hospitalized
   c. child worries
5. a. family member drinks or uses drugs a lot
   b. child worries
6. a. family member has been in trouble with police
   b. child worries
7. a. someone close to child has gotten sick and died
   b. child was very upset
8. a. someone close to child was murdered
   b. child was very upset
   c. someone close to child was killed in an accident
   d. child was very upset
9. anything else we need to know so we can help you?
   _____
   _____
10. problems child thinks he/she needs help with?
    _____
    _____
11. anything in the interview that bothered you?
    _____
    _____

P-ChIPS Report Form

Child's Name: _____ Date: _____ / _____ / _____

Informant's Name: _____ Interviewer: _____

Informant's Relationship (circle one): Mother, Father, Stepmother, Stepfather, Guardian, Other _____

Attention-Deficit/Hyperactivity Disorder

A: Inattention

1. a. pays no attention to details
   b. makes careless mistakes on schoolwork
2. can't keep mind on what he/she is doing
3. a. has trouble listening to parent
   b. has trouble listening to teacher
4. has trouble finishing things
5. has trouble organizing self
6. avoids schoolwork
7. loses school supplies
8. a. is easily distracted
   b. teacher reports inattention/daydreaming
9. a. is forgetful
   b. teacher reports forgetfulness

B: Hyperactivity–Impulsivity

1. a. is often told to sit still
   b. is constantly moving hands/feet
2. a. has trouble staying in seat
   b. gets in trouble for getting out of chair
3. gets in trouble for running/climbing
4. a. is too loud when playing
   b. has difficulty playing quietly
5. teacher reports is always "on the go"
6. a. talks out of turn at school
   b. talks too much at home
7. blurts out answers to questions
8. a. pushes ahead in line
   b. can't wait for his/her turn in games
9. a. barges in on other kids' games
   b. pushes into others' groups
   c. interrupts busy people

Oppositional Defiant Disorder

1. a. loses temper when things don't go his/her way
   b. has frequent temper tantrums
2. a. talks back/argues with parents
   b. talks back/argues with teachers
3. a. breaks rules at home
   b. breaks rules at school
   c. refuses to follow teachers' directions
   d. disobeys direct orders
4. purposely "bugs" other people
5. blames others for his/her own mistakes
6. is easily angered by others
7. is angry a lot of the time
8. gets even when angered

Conduct Disorder

1. has stolen >1 time
2. a. lies to get out of doing things
   b. "cons" people
3. has broken into a car or building to steal
4. has skipped school >3 times
5. breaks curfew >1 time per month
6. has run away/stayed out all night >1 time or did not return for a long time
7. a. is a bully
   b. threatens other people
8. a. is avoided because he/she starts fights
   b. gets in trouble for fighting
9. has used a weapon in a fight >1 time
10. a. has hurt someone badly in a fight
    b. has hurt someone for no reason
11. has taken things from people by force
12. has damaged property
13. has set something on fire (>1 time or caused extensive damage)
14. has hurt or killed an animal for fun
15. a. has forcefully performed sexual activity on another
    b. has forced someone to perform sexual activity on him-/herself

Substance Abuse

1. a. has smoked cigarettes ≥2 times _____
   b. has smoked pot ≥2 times _____
   c. has smoked other drugs ≥2 times _____
2. has used alcohol _____
3. has used other drugs _____
4. has sniffed a substance ≥2 times _____

Specific Phobia

1. phobic object/situation: _____
2. when confronted with object/situation,
   a. gets uptight and scared, can't move
   b. cries, clings to parents, throws tantrums
3. a. avoids object/situation
   b. becomes nauseated, feels faint
4. a. fear interferes with (sleep, school, activities)
   b. feels *super* uncomfortable because of fear
5. a. is more scared of object/situation than peers
   b. fear seems silly to child

Social Phobia

1. a. is afraid of being around other people
   b. has fear of performing
2. feels super-uncomfortable when a/b occurs
3. a. tries to avoid social situations
   b. if unavoidable, feels awful
4. a. fear interferes with (sleep, school, activities)
   b. feels *super* uncomfortable because of fear
5. behavior seems silly to child

Separation Anxiety

1. a. cries, begs parent to stay home
   b. tries to stay home with parent at all times
2. a. worries about parent getting harmed
   b. fears parental harm if separated
3. fears personal harm when separated from parent
4. a. has difficulty going to school
   b. refuses to go to school
5. a. is afraid to be in room of house alone
   b. follows parent around the house
6. a. can't sleep if not with parent
   b. can't sleep away from home
7. a. has nightmares about separation
   b. has nightmares about parental loss
8. a. has stomach- or headaches before going to school
   b. gets ill when parent leaves him/her

Generalized Anxiety Disorder

1. worries more than other kids _____
2. a. has difficulty calming down
   b. can't let go of worry
3. when worried, feels edgy, tired, distractible, cranky; has tight muscles, poor sleep

Obsessive-Compulsive Disorder

A: Compulsions

1. does things over and over
2. a. feels behavior will improve things
   b. thinks that if he/she can't perform behavior, something bad will happen
3. feels that behavior does not make sense

B: Obsessions

1. a. has bothersome thoughts/ideas
   b. "sees" pictures in head repeatedly
   c. has to do something but never does it
2. a. tries to make bothersome thoughts go away
   b. tries to pretend that thoughts aren't there
   c. does other things to try to make thoughts go away

3. thoughts seem like child's own (as opposed to someone else putting thoughts in his/her mind)

C: Interference

1. a. thoughts/behaviors cause child discomfort
   b. thoughts/behaviors cause problems at (home, school, play)
   c. thoughts/behaviors interfere with daily routines (time spent daily: _____)

Stress Disorders—PTSD, ASD

A: Exposure

1. a. child experienced traumatic event _____
   b. child witnessed traumatic event happening to someone else _____
2. after event, felt helpless, shocked, horrified, like he/she was falling apart; was hard to calm down
3. how long ago did event happen? _____

B: Dissociation

1. after event, felt cut off from family/friends; felt fewer emotions, felt numb
2. felt out of touch, in a daze
3. felt that the world was not real
4. felt that self was no longer real
5. had trouble remembering event

C: Reexperiencing

1. a. replays event over and over in mind
   b. "sees" event happening again
   c. plays games about event over and over
2. a. has nightmares about event
   b. has nightmares but can't remember what they're about
3. a. "feels" event happening again
   b. acts like event is happening again
4. a. becomes upset when reminded of event
   b. becomes upset when in same physical setting in which event occurred
5. when reminded of event, gets anxious, achy, sweaty palms, breathing problems

D: Avoidance

1. a. avoids thinking/talking about event
   b. tries to be unafraid of anything
2. a. avoids activities that remind him/her of event
   b. avoids places that remind him/her of event
   c. avoids people that remind him/her of event
3. can't remember things about event
4. a. has decreased interest in things he/she used to enjoy
   b. has stopped doing things he/she used to enjoy
5. feels cut off from family/friends
6. feels fewer emotions; feels numb
7. a. feels he/she won't grow up
   b. feels he/she will die soon

E: Hyperarousal

1. a. has trouble falling asleep
   b. has trouble staying asleep
2. a. is harder to get along with
   b. is easily angered
3. has difficulty concentrating
4. is super-alert
5. is easily startled, jumpy

Anorexia

1. a. has lost weight by dieting
   b. tries to stay underweight
2. a. current weight and height _____
   b. weight and height when thinnest _____
3. a. is terrified of getting fat
   b. is afraid of gaining weight
   c. fears he/she won't stop eating if he/she starts
4. a. feels fat
   b. feels good/bad depending on weight
   c. thinks his/her weight is a problem
5. if she's started menstruation yet, amenorrhea?

Bulimia

1. eats lots of food in short time
2. feels he/she can't stop eating, only stops because
   _____
3. after eating, tries to lose weight by . . .
   a. not eating
   b. vomiting
   c. taking laxatives
   d. overexercising
4. a. is more weight-conscious than peers
   b. self-image depends on weight

Depression/Dysthymia

A: Dysphoric Mood

1. a. feels sad or depressed
   b. almost every day
   c. lasts most of the day
2. a. feels more irritable
   b. (i) fights (ii) cries (iii) temper
   c. almost every day
   d. lasts most of the day

B: Loss of Interest

1. a. used to have fun doing _____
   b. isn't fun anymore
2. a. wants to have fun but can't
   b. feels that nothing is fun anymore
   c. has lost interest in daily activities

C: Appetite Changes

1. a. has decreased appetite
   b. has lost weight without dieting
   c. clothes are too big now
2. a. has increased appetite
   b. has gained weight

D: Sleep Changes

1. goes to bed @ _____; wakes @ _____
   a. early insomnia
   b. middle insomnia
   c. late insomnia
2. a. naps a lot
   b. hypersomnia

E: Psychomotor Changes

1. a. can't sit still
   b. is fidgety
   c. wrings hands
   d. picks at him-/herself
2. a. takes longer to do things
   b. has difficulty doing anything

F: Low Energy

1. a. has no energy
   b. has to push self
   c. tires easily
   d. sits around, does nothing

G: Guilt

1. a. has bad thoughts about self
   b. feels down on self
   c. feels he/she is no good
   d. hates self
2. a. feels guilty a lot
   b. thinks he/she should be punished

H: Impaired Concentration

1. a. mind has slowed down
   b. forgets things more
   c. has trouble paying attention
   d. listens to teacher less than before
   e. grades have dropped
2. has difficulty making up mind

I: Hopelessness

1. a. feels that nothing good will happen in the future
   b. feels that things won't get any better
   c. feels that there's no hope for the future

J: Morbid/Suicidal Thoughts

1. a. thinks about death
   b. thinks about dead people/pets
2. a. wishes he/she were dead
   b. feels life isn't worth living
   c. has thought of suicide
   d. has thought of suicide plans
   e. has made suicide attempt

Mania/Hypomania

A: Elevated Mood

1. a. feels very, very good
   b. feels wonderful for no reason
   c. is "too high"
2. has discrete periods of irritability

B: Other Symptoms

1. a. believes he/she has special abilities
   b. believes he/she can do things better than anyone
2. a. has lots of energy, no need for sleep
   b. sleeps a lot less without feeling tired
   c. needs ≤3 hours of sleep to feel OK
3. a. has rapid, unstoppable speech
   b. talks so fast that family/friends worry
   c. is told he/she talks too much, too loudly
   d. talks too fast to be understood
4. a. thoughts race through mind
   b. thoughts come too fast to verbalize them all
   c. feels that mind is sped up, working too fast
5. has trouble focusing
6. a. does more things than usual
   b. has more energy than usual
   c. tries many different things
   d. family/friends are concerned
   e. is more active than usual
7. a. gets in trouble more
   b. does things he/she usually wouldn't
   c. gets hurt due to carelessness
   d. is a lot more interested in sex than usual

C: Interference

1. mood/behavior causes problems at (home, school, play)
2. mood/behavior is reason child is here

Enuresis

1. has wet bed after kindergarten
2. a. wets bed at night
   b. wets self during day
3. a. occurs when not sick
   b. is not due to effects of some medication

Encopresis

1. has had bowel movement outside of toilet after kindergarten
2. happens when not sick

Schizophrenia/Psychosis

A: Psychotic Symptoms

1. a. feels someone is out to harm him/her
   b. feels someone is trying to make him/her sick
   c. people seem to be against him/her
   d. people seem to talk about him/her
   e. people spy on him/her
2. a. eyes play tricks on him/her
   b. during daylight
   c. only when falling asleep
   d. ears play tricks on him/her
   e. voices talk about child's feelings/thoughts/acts
   f. voices talk to each other

Interviewer observed:
3. *incoherent speech*
4. *disorganized or catatonic behavior*
5. *inappropriate affect or inability to speak*

B: Interference

1. since problems started, has more difficulty getting along with other people
2. since problems started, does worse in school
3. since problems started, is careless about looks/ hygiene

Psychosocial Stressors

A: Child Abuse/Neglect

1. a. M/F criticizes child a lot
   b. M/F wishes child had never been born
   c. M/F says he/she hates child
2. a. M/F ignores child
   b. M/F misses child's doctor appointments
   c. M/F does not feed child
   d. M/F does not clothe child
3. a. child is spanked or hit
   b. child is sometimes spanked or hit for no reason
   c. child fears physical harm from M/F
   d. child has been bruised, sore, taken to doctor
4. child has been sexually abused
5. child has been made to go a whole day without food

B: Other Stressors

1. a. fighting within family
   b. among children
   c. between parents
   d. between parents and children
   e. fighting bothers child
2. child remembers parents' separation/divorce
3. a. family has money problems
   b. child is worried about money problems
4. a. family member is ill
   b. family member has been hospitalized
   c. child worries
5. a. family member drinks or uses drugs a lot
   b. child worries
6. a. family member has been in trouble with police
   b. child worries
7. a. someone close to child has gotten sick and died
   b. child was very upset
8. a. someone close to child was murdered
   b. child was very upset
   c. someone close to child was killed in an accident
   d. child was very upset
9. anything else we need to know so we can help you?
   _____
   _____
10. problems child thinks he/she needs help with?
    _____
    _____
11. anything in the interview that bothered you?
    _____
    _____

P-ChIPS Report Form

Child's Name: _____ Date: _____ / _____ / _____

Informant's Name: _____ Interviewer: _____

Informant's Relationship (circle one): Mother, Father, Stepmother, Stepfather, Guardian, Other _____

Attention-Deficit/Hyperactivity Disorder

A: Inattention

1. a. pays no attention to details
   b. makes careless mistakes on schoolwork
2. can't keep mind on what he/she is doing
3. a. has trouble listening to parent
   b. has trouble listening to teacher
4. has trouble finishing things
5. has trouble organizing self
6. avoids schoolwork
7. loses school supplies
8. a. is easily distracted
   b. teacher reports inattention/daydreaming
9. a. is forgetful
   b. teacher reports forgetfulness

B: Hyperactivity–Impulsivity

1. a. is often told to sit still
   b. is constantly moving hands/feet
2. a. has trouble staying in seat
   b. gets in trouble for getting out of chair
3. gets in trouble for running/climbing
4. a. is too loud when playing
   b. has difficulty playing quietly
5. teacher reports is always "on the go"
6. a. talks out of turn at school
   b. talks too much at home
7. blurts out answers to questions
8. a. pushes ahead in line
   b. can't wait for his/her turn in games
9. a. barges in on other kids' games
   b. pushes into others' groups
   c. interrupts busy people

Oppositional Defiant Disorder

1. a. loses temper when things don't go his/her way
   b. has frequent temper tantrums
2. a. talks back/argues with parents
   b. talks back/argues with teachers
3. a. breaks rules at home
   b. breaks rules at school
   c. refuses to follow teachers' directions
   d. disobeys direct orders
4. purposely "bugs" other people
5. blames others for his/her own mistakes
6. is easily angered by others
7. is angry a lot of the time
8. gets even when angered

Conduct Disorder

1. has stolen >1 time
2. a. lies to get out of doing things
   b. "cons" people
3. has broken into a car or building to steal
4. has skipped school >3 times
5. breaks curfew >1 time per month
6. has run away/stayed out all night >1 time *or* did not return for a long time
7. a. is a bully
   b. threatens other people
8. a. is avoided because he/she starts fights
   b. gets in trouble for fighting
9. has used a weapon in a fight >1 time
10. a. has hurt someone badly in a fight
    b. has hurt someone for no reason
11. has taken things from people by force
12. has damaged property
13. has set something on fire (>1 time *or* caused extensive damage)
14. has hurt or killed an animal for fun
15. a. has forcefully performed sexual activity on another
    b. has forced someone to perform sexual activity on him-/herself

Substance Abuse

1. a. has smoked cigarettes ≥2 times _____
   b. has smoked pot ≥2 times _____
   c. has smoked other drugs ≥2 times _____
2. has used alcohol _____
3. has used other drugs _____
4. has sniffed a substance ≥2 times _____

Specific Phobia

1. phobic object/situation: _____
2. when confronted with object/situation,
    a. gets uptight and scared, can't move
    b. cries, clings to parents, throws tantrums
3. a. avoids object/situation
    b. becomes nauseated, feels faint
4. a. fear interferes with (sleep, school, activities)
    b. feels *super* uncomfortable because of fear
5. a. is more scared of object/situation than peers
    b. fear seems silly to child

Social Phobia

1. a. is afraid of being around other people
    b. has fear of performing
2. feels super-uncomfortable when a/b occurs
3. a. tries to avoid social situations
    b. if unavoidable, feels awful
4. a. fear interferes with (sleep, school, activities)
    b. feels *super* uncomfortable because of fear
5. behavior seems silly to child

Separation Anxiety

1. a. cries, begs parent to stay home
    b. tries to stay home with parent at all times
2. a. worries about parent getting harmed
    b. fears parental harm if separated
3. fears personal harm when separated from parent
4. a. has difficulty going to school
    b. refuses to go to school
5. a. is afraid to be in room of house alone
    b. follows parent around the house
6. a. can't sleep if not with parent
    b. can't sleep away from home
7. a. has nightmares about separation
    b. has nightmares about parental loss
8. a. has stomach- or headaches before going to school
    b. gets ill when parent leaves him/her

Generalized Anxiety Disorder

1. worries more than other kids _____
2. a. has difficulty calming down
    b. can't let go of worry
3. when worried, feels edgy, tired, distractible, cranky; has tight muscles, poor sleep

Obsessive-Compulsive Disorder

A: Compulsions

1. does things over and over
2. a. feels behavior will improve things
    b. thinks that if he/she can't perform behavior, something bad will happen
3. feels that behavior does not make sense

B: Obsessions

1. a. has bothersome thoughts/ideas
    b. "sees" pictures in head repeatedly
    c. has to do something but never does it
2. a. tries to make bothersome thoughts go away
    b. tries to pretend that thoughts aren't there
    c. does other things to try to make thoughts go away

3. thoughts seem like child's own (as opposed to someone else putting thoughts in his/her mind)

C: Interference

1. a. thoughts/behaviors cause child discomfort
    b. thoughts/behaviors cause problems at (home, school, play)
    c. thoughts/behaviors interfere with daily routines (time spent daily: _____)

Stress Disorders—PTSD, ASD

A: Exposure

1. a. child experienced traumatic event _____
    b. child witnessed traumatic event happening to someone else _____
2. after event, felt helpless, shocked, horrified, like he/she was falling apart; was hard to calm down
3. how long ago did event happen? _____

B: Dissociation

1. after event, felt cut off from family/friends; felt fewer emotions, felt numb
2. felt out of touch, in a daze
3. felt that the world was not real
4. felt that self was no longer real
5. had trouble remembering event

C: Reexperiencing

1. a. replays event over and over in mind
    b. "sees" event happening again
    c. plays games about event over and over
2. a. has nightmares about event
    b. has nightmares but can't remember what they're about
3. a. "feels" event happening again
    b. acts like event is happening again
4. a. becomes upset when reminded of event
    b. becomes upset when in same physical setting in which event occurred
5. when reminded of event, gets anxious, achy, sweaty palms, breathing problems

D: Avoidance

1. a. avoids thinking/talking about event
    b. tries to be unafraid of anything
2. a. avoids activities that remind him/her of event
    b. avoids places that remind him/her of event
    c. avoids people that remind him/her of event
3. can't remember things about event
4. a. has decreased interest in things he/she used to enjoy
    b. has stopped doing things he/she used to enjoy
5. feels cut off from family/friends
6. feels fewer emotions; feels numb
7. a. feels he/she won't grow up
    b. feels he/she will die soon

E: Hyperarousal

1. a. has trouble falling asleep
    b. has trouble staying asleep
2. a. is harder to get along with
    b. is easily angered
3. has difficulty concentrating
4. is super-alert
5. is easily startled, jumpy

Anorexia

1. a. has lost weight by dieting
   b. tries to stay underweight
2. a. current weight and height _____
   b. weight and height when thinnest _____
3. a. is terrified of getting fat
   b. is afraid of gaining weight
   c. fears he/she won't stop eating if he/she starts
4. a. feels fat
   b. feels good/bad depending on weight
   c. thinks his/her weight is a problem
5. if she's started menstruation yet, amenorrhea?

Bulimia

1. eats lots of food in short time
2. feels he/she can't stop eating, only stops because
   _____
3. after eating, tries to lose weight by . . .
   a. not eating
   b. vomiting
   c. taking laxatives
   d. overexercising
4. a. is more weight-conscious than peers
   b. self-image depends on weight

Depression/Dysthymia

A: Dysphoric Mood
1. a. feels sad or depressed
   b. almost every day
   c. lasts most of the day
2. a. feels more irritable
   b. (i) fights (ii) cries (iii) temper
   c. almost every day
   d. lasts most of the day

B: Loss of Interest
1. a. used to have fun doing _____
   b. isn't fun anymore
2. a. wants to have fun but can't
   b. feels that nothing is fun anymore
   c. has lost interest in daily activities

C: Appetite Changes
1. a. has decreased appetite
   b. has lost weight without dieting
   c. clothes are too big now
2. a. has increased appetite
   b. has gained weight

D: Sleep Changes
1. goes to bed @ _____; wakes @ _____
   a. early insomnia
   b. middle insomnia
   c. late insomnia
2. a. naps a lot
   b. hypersomnia

E: Psychomotor Changes
1. a. can't sit still
   b. is fidgety
   c. wrings hands
   d. picks at him-/herself
2. a. takes longer to do things
   b. has difficulty doing anything

F: Low Energy
1. a. has no energy
   b. has to push self
   c. tires easily
   d. sits around, does nothing

G: Guilt
1. a. has bad thoughts about self
   b. feels down on self
   c. feels he/she is no good
   d. hates self
2. a. feels guilty a lot
   b. thinks he/she should be punished

H: Impaired Concentration
1. a. mind has slowed down
   b. forgets things more
   c. has trouble paying attention
   d. listens to teacher less than before
   e. grades have dropped
2. has difficulty making up mind

I: Hopelessness
1. a. feels that nothing good will happen in the future
   b. feels that things won't get any better
   c. feels that there's no hope for the future

J: Morbid/Suicidal Thoughts
1. a. thinks about death
   b. thinks about dead people/pets
2. a. wishes he/she were dead
   b. feels life isn't worth living
   c. has thought of suicide
   d. has thought of suicide plans
   e. has made suicide attempt

Mania/Hypomania

A: Elevated Mood
1. a. feels very, very good
   b. feels wonderful for no reason
   c. is "too high"
2. has discrete periods of irritability

B: Other Symptoms
1. a. believes he/she has special abilities
   b. believes he/she can do things better than anyone
2. a. has lots of energy, no need for sleep
   b. sleeps a lot less without feeling tired
   c. needs ≤3 hours of sleep to feel OK
3. a. has rapid, unstoppable speech
   b. talks so fast that family/friends worry
   c. is told he/she talks too much, too loudly
   d. talks too fast to be understood
4. a. thoughts race through mind
   b. thoughts come too fast to verbalize them all
   c. feels that mind is sped up, working too fast
5. has trouble focusing
6. a. does more things than usual
   b. has more energy than usual
   c. tries many different things
   d. family/friends are concerned
   e. is more active than usual
7. a. gets in trouble more
   b. does things he/she usually wouldn't
   c. gets hurt due to carelessness
   d. is a lot more interested in sex than usual

C: Interference
1. mood/behavior causes problems at (home, school, play)
2. mood/behavior is reason child is here

Enuresis

1. has wet bed after kindergarten
2. a. wets bed at night
   b. wets self during day
3. a. occurs when not sick
   b. is not due to effects of some medication

Encopresis

1. has had bowel movement outside of toilet after kindergarten
2. happens when not sick

Schizophrenia/Psychosis

A: Psychotic Symptoms

1. a. feels someone is out to harm him/her
   b. feels someone is trying to make him/her sick
   c. people seem to be against him/her
   d. people seem to talk about him/her
   e. people spy on him/her
2. a. eyes play tricks on him/her
   b. during daylight
   c. only when falling asleep
   d. ears play tricks on him/her
   e. voices talk about child's feelings/thoughts/acts
   f. voices talk to each other

Interviewer observed:
3. *incoherent speech*
4. *disorganized or catatonic behavior*
5. *inappropriate affect or inability to speak*

B: Interference

1. since problems started, has more difficulty getting along with other people
2. since problems started, does worse in school
3. since problems started, is careless about looks/ hygiene

Psychosocial Stressors

A: Child Abuse/Neglect

1. a. M/F criticizes child a lot
   b. M/F wishes child had never been born
   c. M/F says he/she hates child
2. a. M/F ignores child
   b. M/F misses child's doctor appointments
   c. M/F does not feed child
   d. M/F does not clothe child
3. a. child is spanked or hit
   b. child is sometimes spanked or hit for no reason
   c. child fears physical harm from M/F
   d. child has been bruised, sore, taken to doctor
4. child has been sexually abused
5. child has been made to go a whole day without food

B: Other Stressors

1. a. fighting within family
   b. among children
   c. between parents
   d. between parents and children
   e. fighting bothers child
2. child remembers parents' separation/divorce
3. a. family has money problems
   b. child is worried about money problems
4. a. family member is ill
   b. family member has been hospitalized
   c. child worries
5. a. family member drinks or uses drugs a lot
   b. child worries
6. a. family member has been in trouble with police
   b. child worries
7. a. someone close to child has gotten sick and died
   b. child was very upset
8. a. someone close to child was murdered
   b. child was very upset
   c. someone close to child was killed in an accident
   d. child was very upset
9. anything else we need to know so we can help you?

   _____
   _____

10. problems child thinks he/she needs help with?

    _____
    _____

11. anything in the interview that bothered you?

    _____
    _____

P-ChIPS Report Form

Child's Name: _____ Date: _____ / _____ / _____

Informant's Name: _____ Interviewer: _____

Informant's Relationship (circle one): Mother, Father, Stepmother, Stepfather, Guardian, Other _____

Attention-Deficit/Hyperactivity Disorder

A: Inattention

1. a. pays no attention to details
   b. makes careless mistakes on schoolwork
2. can't keep mind on what he/she is doing
3. a. has trouble listening to parent
   b. has trouble listening to teacher
4. has trouble finishing things
5. has trouble organizing self
6. avoids schoolwork
7. loses school supplies
8. a. is easily distracted
   b. teacher reports inattention/daydreaming
9. a. is forgetful
   b. teacher reports forgetfulness

B: Hyperactivity–Impulsivity

1. a. is often told to sit still
   b. is constantly moving hands/feet
2. a. has trouble staying in seat
   b. gets in trouble for getting out of chair
3. gets in trouble for running/climbing
4. a. is too loud when playing
   b. has difficulty playing quietly
5. teacher reports is always "on the go"
6. a. talks out of turn at school
   b. talks too much at home
7. blurts out answers to questions
8. a. pushes ahead in line
   b. can't wait for his/her turn in games
9. a. barges in on other kids' games
   b. pushes into others' groups
   c. interrupts busy people

Oppositional Defiant Disorder

1. a. loses temper when things don't go his/her way
   b. has frequent temper tantrums
2. a. talks back/argues with parents
   b. talks back/argues with teachers
3. a. breaks rules at home
   b. breaks rules at school
   c. refuses to follow teachers' directions
   d. disobeys direct orders
4. purposely "bugs" other people
5. blames others for his/her own mistakes
6. is easily angered by others
7. is angry a lot of the time
8. gets even when angered

Conduct Disorder

1. has stolen >1 time
2. a. lies to get out of doing things
   b. "cons" people
3. has broken into a car or building to steal
4. has skipped school >3 times
5. breaks curfew >1 time per month
6. has run away/stayed out all night >1 time *or* did not return for a long time
7. a. is a bully
   b. threatens other people
8. a. is avoided because he/she starts fights
   b. gets in trouble for fighting
9. has used a weapon in a fight >1 time
10. a. has hurt someone badly in a fight
    b. has hurt someone for no reason
11. has taken things from people by force
12. has damaged property
13. has set something on fire (>1 time *or* caused extensive damage)
14. has hurt or killed an animal for fun
15. a. has forcefully performed sexual activity on another
    b. has forced someone to perform sexual activity on him-/herself

Substance Abuse

1. a. has smoked cigarettes ≥2 times _____
   b. has smoked pot ≥2 times _____
   c. has smoked other drugs ≥2 times _____
2. has used alcohol _____
3. has used other drugs _____
4. has sniffed a substance ≥2 times _____

Specific Phobia

1. phobic object/situation: _____
2. when confronted with object/situation,
   a. gets uptight and scared, can't move
   b. cries, clings to parents, throws tantrums
3. a. avoids object/situation
   b. becomes nauseated, feels faint
4. a. fear interferes with (sleep, school, activities)
   b. feels *super* uncomfortable because of fear
5. a. is more scared of object/situation than peers
   b. fear seems silly to child

Social Phobia

1. a. is afraid of being around other people
   b. has fear of performing
2. feels super-uncomfortable when a/b occurs
3. a. tries to avoid social situations
   b. if unavoidable, feels awful
4. a. fear interferes with (sleep, school, activities)
   b. feels *super* uncomfortable because of fear
5. behavior seems silly to child

Separation Anxiety

1. a. cries, begs parent to stay home
   b. tries to stay home with parent at all times
2. a. worries about parent getting harmed
   b. fears parental harm if separated
3. fears personal harm when separated from parent
4. a. has difficulty going to school
   b. refuses to go to school
5. a. is afraid to be in room of house alone
   b. follows parent around the house
6. a. can't sleep if not with parent
   b. can't sleep away from home
7. a. has nightmares about separation
   b. has nightmares about parental loss
8. a. has stomach- or headaches before going to school
   b. gets ill when parent leaves him/her

Generalized Anxiety Disorder

1. worries more than other kids _____
2. a. has difficulty calming down
   b. can't let go of worry
3. when worried, feels edgy, tired, distractible, cranky; has tight muscles, poor sleep

Obsessive-Compulsive Disorder

A: Compulsions

1. does things over and over
2. a. feels behavior will improve things
   b. thinks that if he/she can't perform behavior, something bad will happen
3. feels that behavior does not make sense

B: Obsessions

1. a. has bothersome thoughts/ideas
   b. "sees" pictures in head repeatedly
   c. has to do something but never does it
2. a. tries to make bothersome thoughts go away
   b. tries to pretend that thoughts aren't there
   c. does other things to try to make thoughts go away

3. thoughts seem like child's own (as opposed to someone else putting thoughts in his/her mind)

C: Interference

1. a. thoughts/behaviors cause child discomfort
   b. thoughts/behaviors cause problems at (home, school, play)
   c. thoughts/behaviors interfere with daily routines (time spent daily: _____)

Stress Disorders—PTSD, ASD

A: Exposure

1. a. child experienced traumatic event _____
   b. child witnessed traumatic event happening to someone else _____
2. after event, felt helpless, shocked, horrified, like he/she was falling apart; was hard to calm down
3. how long ago did event happen? _____

B: Dissociation

1. after event, felt cut off from family/friends; felt fewer emotions, felt numb
2. felt out of touch, in a daze
3. felt that the world was not real
4. felt that self was no longer real
5. had trouble remembering event

C: Reexperiencing

1. a. replays event over and over in mind
   b. "sees" event happening again
   c. plays games about event over and over
2. a. has nightmares about event
   b. has nightmares but can't remember what they're about
3. a. "feels" event happening again
   b. acts like event is happening again
4. a. becomes upset when reminded of event
   b. becomes upset when in same physical setting in which event occurred
5. when reminded of event, gets anxious, achy, sweaty palms, breathing problems

D: Avoidance

1. a. avoids thinking/talking about event
   b. tries to be unafraid of anything
2. a. avoids activities that remind him/her of event
   b. avoids places that remind him/her of event
   c. avoids people that remind him/her of event
3. can't remember things about event
4. a. has decreased interest in things he/she used to enjoy
   b. has stopped doing things he/she used to enjoy
5. feels cut off from family/friends
6. feels fewer emotions; feels numb
7. a. feels he/she won't grow up
   b. feels he/she will die soon

E: Hyperarousal

1. a. has trouble falling asleep
   b. has trouble staying asleep
2. a. is harder to get along with
   b. is easily angered
3. has difficulty concentrating
4. is super-alert
5. is easily startled, jumpy

Anorexia

1. a. has lost weight by dieting
   b. tries to stay underweight
2. a. current weight and height _____
   b. weight and height when thinnest _____
3. a. is terrified of getting fat
   b. is afraid of gaining weight
   c. fears he/she won't stop eating if he/she starts
4. a. feels fat
   b. feels good/bad depending on weight
   c. thinks his/her weight is a problem
5. if she's started menstruation yet, amenorrhea?

Bulimia

1. eats lots of food in short time
2. feels he/she can't stop eating, only stops because
   _____
3. after eating, tries to lose weight by . . .
   a. not eating
   b. vomiting
   c. taking laxatives
   d. overexercising
4. a. is more weight-conscious than peers
   b. self-image depends on weight

Depression/Dysthymia

A: Dysphoric Mood
1. a. feels sad or depressed
   b. almost every day
   c. lasts most of the day
2. a. feels more irritable
   b. (i) fights (ii) cries (iii) temper
   c. almost every day
   d. lasts most of the day

B: Loss of Interest
1. a. used to have fun doing _____
   b. isn't fun anymore
2. a. wants to have fun but can't
   b. feels that nothing is fun anymore
   c. has lost interest in daily activities

C: Appetite Changes
1. a. has decreased appetite
   b. has lost weight without dieting
   c. clothes are too big now
2. a. has increased appetite
   b. has gained weight

D: Sleep Changes
1. goes to bed @ _____; wakes @ _____
   a. early insomnia
   b. middle insomnia
   c. late insomnia
2. a. naps a lot
   b. hypersomnia

E: Psychomotor Changes
1. a. can't sit still
   b. is fidgety
   c. wrings hands
   d. picks at him-/herself
2. a. takes longer to do things
   b. has difficulty doing anything

F: Low Energy
1. a. has no energy
   b. has to push self
   c. tires easily
   d. sits around, does nothing

G: Guilt
1. a. has bad thoughts about self
   b. feels down on self
   c. feels he/she is no good
   d. hates self
2. a. feels guilty a lot
   b. thinks he/she should be punished

H: Impaired Concentration
1. a. mind has slowed down
   b. forgets things more
   c. has trouble paying attention
   d. listens to teacher less than before
   e. grades have dropped
2. has difficulty making up mind

I: Hopelessness
1. a. feels that nothing good will happen in the future
   b. feels that things won't get any better
   c. feels that there's no hope for the future

J: Morbid/Suicidal Thoughts
1. a. thinks about death
   b. thinks about dead people/pets
2. a. wishes he/she were dead
   b. feels life isn't worth living
   c. has thought of suicide
   d. has thought of suicide plans
   e. has made suicide attempt

Mania/Hypomania

A: Elevated Mood
1. a. feels very, very good
   b. feels wonderful for no reason
   c. is "too high"
2. has discrete periods of irritability

B: Other Symptoms
1. a. believes he/she has special abilities
   b. believes he/she can do things better than anyone
2. a. has lots of energy, no need for sleep
   b. sleeps a lot less without feeling tired
   c. needs ≤3 hours of sleep to feel OK
3. a. has rapid, unstoppable speech
   b. talks so fast that family/friends worry
   c. is told he/she talks too much, too loudly
   d. talks too fast to be understood
4. a. thoughts race through mind
   b. thoughts come too fast to verbalize them all
   c. feels that mind is sped up, working too fast
5. has trouble focusing
6. a. does more things than usual
   b. has more energy than usual
   c. tries many different things
   d. family/friends are concerned
   e. is more active than usual
7. a. gets in trouble more
   b. does things he/she usually wouldn't
   c. gets hurt due to carelessness
   d. is a lot more interested in sex than usual

C: Interference
1. mood/behavior causes problems at (home, school, play)
2. mood/behavior is reason child is here

Enuresis

1. has wet bed after kindergarten
2. a. wets bed at night
   b. wets self during day
3. a. occurs when not sick
   b. is not due to effects of some medication

Encopresis

1. has had bowel movement outside of toilet after kindergarten
2. happens when not sick

Schizophrenia/Psychosis

A: Psychotic Symptoms

1. a. feels someone is out to harm him/her
   b. feels someone is trying to make him/her sick
   c. people seem to be against him/her
   d. people seem to talk about him/her
   e. people spy on him/her
2. a. eyes play tricks on him/her
   b. during daylight
   c. only when falling asleep
   d. ears play tricks on him/her
   e. voices talk about child's feelings/thoughts/acts
   f. voices talk to each other

> **Interviewer observed:**
> 3. incoherent speech
> 4. disorganized or catatonic behavior
> 5. inappropriate affect or inability to speak

B: Interference

1. since problems started, has more difficulty getting along with other people
2. since problems started, does worse in school
3. since problems started, is careless about looks/hygiene

Psychosocial Stressors

A: Child Abuse/Neglect

1. a. M/F criticizes child a lot
   b. M/F wishes child had never been born
   c. M/F says he/she hates child
2. a. M/F ignores child
   b. M/F misses child's doctor appointments
   c. M/F does not feed child
   d. M/F does not clothe child
3. a. child is spanked or hit
   b. child is sometimes spanked or hit for no reason
   c. child fears physical harm from M/F
   d. child has been bruised, sore, taken to doctor
4. child has been sexually abused
5. child has been made to go a whole day without food

B: Other Stressors

1. a. fighting within family
   b. among children
   c. between parents
   d. between parents and children
   e. fighting bothers child
2. child remembers parents' separation/divorce
3. a. family has money problems
   b. child is worried about money problems
4. a. family member is ill
   b. family member has been hospitalized
   c. child worries
5. a. family member drinks or uses drugs a lot
   b. child worries
6. a. family member has been in trouble with police
   b. child worries
7. a. someone close to child has gotten sick and died
   b. child was very upset
8. a. someone close to child was murdered
   b. child was very upset
   c. someone close to child was killed in an accident
   d. child was very upset
9. anything else we need to know so we can help you?
   _____
   _____
10. problems child thinks he/she needs help with?
    _____
    _____
11. anything in the interview that bothered you?
    _____
    _____

P-ChIPS Report Form

Child's Name: _____ Date: ____ / _____ / _____

Informant's Name: _____ Interviewer: _____

Informant's Relationship (circle one): Mother, Father, Stepmother, Stepfather, Guardian, Other _____

Attention-Deficit/Hyperactivity Disorder

A: Inattention

1. a. pays no attention to details
   b. makes careless mistakes on schoolwork
2. can't keep mind on what he/she is doing
3. a. has trouble listening to parent
   b. has trouble listening to teacher
4. has trouble finishing things
5. has trouble organizing self
6. avoids schoolwork
7. loses school supplies
8. a. is easily distracted
   b. teacher reports inattention/daydreaming
9. a. is forgetful
   b. teacher reports forgetfulness

B: Hyperactivity–Impulsivity

1. a. is often told to sit still
   b. is constantly moving hands/feet
2. a. has trouble staying in seat
   b. gets in trouble for getting out of chair
3. gets in trouble for running/climbing
4. a. is too loud when playing
   b. has difficulty playing quietly
5. teacher reports is always "on the go"
6. a. talks out of turn at school
   b. talks too much at home
7. blurts out answers to questions
8. a. pushes ahead in line
   b. can't wait for his/her turn in games
9. a. barges in on other kids' games
   b. pushes into others' groups
   c. interrupts busy people

Oppositional Defiant Disorder

1. a. loses temper when things don't go his/her way
   b. has frequent temper tantrums
2. a. talks back/argues with parents
   b. talks back/argues with teachers
3. a. breaks rules at home
   b. breaks rules at school
   c. refuses to follow teachers' directions
   d. disobeys direct orders
4. purposely "bugs" other people
5. blames others for his/her own mistakes
6. is easily angered by others
7. is angry a lot of the time
8. gets even when angered

Conduct Disorder

1. has stolen >1 time
2. a. lies to get out of doing things
   b. "cons" people
3. has broken into a car or building to steal
4. has skipped school >3 times
5. breaks curfew >1 time per month
6. has run away/stayed out all night >1 time *or* did not return for a long time
7. a. is a bully
   b. threatens other people
8. a. is avoided because he/she starts fights
   b. gets in trouble for fighting
9. has used a weapon in a fight >1 time
10. a. has hurt someone badly in a fight
    b. has hurt someone for no reason
11. has taken things from people by force
12. has damaged property
13. has set something on fire (>1 time *or* caused extensive damage)
14. has hurt or killed an animal for fun
15. a. has forcefully performed sexual activity on another
    b. has forced someone to perform sexual activity on him-/herself

Substance Abuse

1. a. has smoked cigarettes ≥2 times _____
   b. has smoked pot ≥2 times _____
   c. has smoked other drugs ≥2 times _____
2. has used alcohol _____
3. has used other drugs _____
4. has sniffed a substance ≥2 times _____

Specific Phobia

1. phobic object/situation: _____
2. when confronted with object/situation,
   a. gets uptight and scared, can't move
   b. cries, clings to parents, throws tantrums
3. a. avoids object/situation
   b. becomes nauseated, feels faint
4. a. fear interferes with (sleep, school, activities)
   b. feels *super* uncomfortable because of fear
5. a. is more scared of object/situation than peers
   b. fear seems silly to child

Social Phobia

1. a. is afraid of being around other people
   b. has fear of performing
2. feels super-uncomfortable when a/b occurs
3. a. tries to avoid social situations
   b. if unavoidable, feels awful
4. a. fear interferes with (sleep, school, activities)
   b. feels *super* uncomfortable because of fear
5. behavior seems silly to child

Separation Anxiety

1. a. cries, begs parent to stay home
   b. tries to stay home with parent at all times
2. a. worries about parent getting harmed
   b. fears parental harm if separated
3. fears personal harm when separated from parent
4. a. has difficulty going to school
   b. refuses to go to school
5. a. is afraid to be in room of house alone
   b. follows parent around the house
6. a. can't sleep if not with parent
   b. can't sleep away from home
7. a. has nightmares about separation
   b. has nightmares about parental loss
8. a. has stomach- or headaches before going to school
   b. gets ill when parent leaves him/her

Generalized Anxiety Disorder

1. worries more than other kids _____
2. a. has difficulty calming down
   b. can't let go of worry
3. when worried, feels edgy, tired, distractible, cranky; has tight muscles, poor sleep

Obsessive-Compulsive Disorder

A: Compulsions

1. does things over and over
2. a. feels behavior will improve things
   b. thinks that if he/she can't perform behavior, something bad will happen
3. feels that behavior does not make sense

B: Obsessions

1. a. has bothersome thoughts/ideas
   b. "sees" pictures in head repeatedly
   c. has to do something but never does it
2. a. tries to make bothersome thoughts go away
   b. tries to pretend that thoughts aren't there
   c. does other things to try to make thoughts go away

3. thoughts seem like child's own (as opposed to someone else putting thoughts in his/her mind)

C: Interference

1. a. thoughts/behaviors cause child discomfort
   b. thoughts/behaviors cause problems at (home, school, play)
   c. thoughts/behaviors interfere with daily routines (time spent daily: _____)

Stress Disorders—PTSD, ASD

A: Exposure

1. a. child experienced traumatic event _____
   b. child witnessed traumatic event happening to someone else _____
2. after event, felt helpless, shocked, horrified, like he/she was falling apart; was hard to calm down
3. how long ago did event happen? _____

B: Dissociation

1. after event, felt cut off from family/friends; felt fewer emotions, felt numb
2. felt out of touch, in a daze
3. felt that the world was not real
4. felt that self was no longer real
5. had trouble remembering event

C: Reexperiencing

1. a. replays event over and over in mind
   b. "sees" event happening again
   c. plays games about event over and over
2. a. has nightmares about event
   b. has nightmares but can't remember what they're about
3. a. "feels" event happening again
   b. acts like event is happening again
4. a. becomes upset when reminded of event
   b. becomes upset when in same physical setting in which event occurred
5. when reminded of event, gets anxious, achy, sweaty palms, breathing problems

D: Avoidance

1. a. avoids thinking/talking about event
   b. tries to be unafraid of anything
2. a. avoids activities that remind him/her of event
   b. avoids places that remind him/her of event
   c. avoids people that remind him/her of event
3. can't remember things about event
4. a. has decreased interest in things he/she used to enjoy
   b. has stopped doing things he/she used to enjoy
5. feels cut off from family/friends
6. feels fewer emotions; feels numb
7. a. feels he/she won't grow up
   b. feels he/she will die soon

E: Hyperarousal

1. a. has trouble falling asleep
   b. has trouble staying asleep
2. a. is harder to get along with
   b. is easily angered
3. has difficulty concentrating
4. is super-alert
5. is easily startled, jumpy

Anorexia

1. a. has lost weight by dieting
   b. tries to stay underweight
2. a. current weight and height _____
   b. weight and height when thinnest _____
3. a. is terrified of getting fat
   b. is afraid of gaining weight
   c. fears he/she won't stop eating if he/she starts
4. a. feels fat
   b. feels good/bad depending on weight
   c. thinks his/her weight is a problem
5. if she's started menstruation yet, amenorrhea?

Bulimia

1. eats lots of food in short time
2. feels he/she can't stop eating, only stops because
   _____
3. after eating, tries to lose weight by . . .
   a. not eating
   b. vomiting
   c. taking laxatives
   d. overexercising
4. a. is more weight-conscious than peers
   b. self-image depends on weight

Depression/Dysthymia

A: Dysphoric Mood

1. a. feels sad or depressed
   b. almost every day
   c. lasts most of the day
2. a. feels more irritable
   b. (i) fights (ii) cries (iii) temper
   c. almost every day
   d. lasts most of the day

B: Loss of Interest

1. a. used to have fun doing _____
   b. isn't fun anymore
2. a. wants to have fun but can't
   b. feels that nothing is fun anymore
   c. has lost interest in daily activities

C: Appetite Changes

1. a. has decreased appetite
   b. has lost weight without dieting
   c. clothes are too big now
2. a. has increased appetite
   b. has gained weight

D: Sleep Changes

1. goes to bed @ _____; wakes @ _____
   a. early insomnia
   b. middle insomnia
   c. late insomnia
2. a. naps a lot
   b. hypersomnia

E: Psychomotor Changes

1. a. can't sit still
   b. is fidgety
   c. wrings hands
   d. picks at him-/herself
2. a. takes longer to do things
   b. has difficulty doing anything

F: Low Energy

1. a. has no energy
   b. has to push self
   c. tires easily
   d. sits around, does nothing

G: Guilt

1. a. has bad thoughts about self
   b. feels down on self
   c. feels he/she is no good
   d. hates self
2. a. feels guilty a lot
   b. thinks he/she should be punished

H: Impaired Concentration

1. a. mind has slowed down
   b. forgets things more
   c. has trouble paying attention
   d. listens to teacher less than before
   e. grades have dropped
2. has difficulty making up mind

I: Hopelessness

1. a. feels that nothing good will happen in the future
   b. feels that things won't get any better
   c. feels that there's no hope for the future

J: Morbid/Suicidal Thoughts

1. a. thinks about death
   b. thinks about dead people/pets
2. a. wishes he/she were dead
   b. feels life isn't worth living
   c. has thought of suicide
   d. has thought of suicide plans
   e. has made suicide attempt

Mania/Hypomania

A: Elevated Mood

1. a. feels very, very good
   b. feels wonderful for no reason
   c. is "too high"
2. has discrete periods of irritability

B: Other Symptoms

1. a. believes he/she has special abilities
   b. believes he/she can do things better than anyone
2. a. has lots of energy, no need for sleep
   b. sleeps a lot less without feeling tired
   c. needs ≤3 hours of sleep to feel OK
3. a. has rapid, unstoppable speech
   b. talks so fast that family/friends worry
   c. is told he/she talks too much, too loudly
   d. talks too fast to be understood
4. a. thoughts race through mind
   b. thoughts come too fast to verbalize them all
   c. feels that mind is sped up, working too fast
5. has trouble focusing
6. a. does more things than usual
   b. has more energy than usual
   c. tries many different things
   d. family/friends are concerned
   e. is more active than usual
7. a. gets in trouble more
   b. does things he/she usually wouldn't
   c. gets hurt due to carelessness
   d. is a lot more interested in sex than usual

C: Interference

1. mood/behavior causes problems at (home, school, play)
2. mood/behavior is reason child is here

Enuresis

1. has wet bed after kindergarten
2. a. wets bed at night
   b. wets self during day
3. a. occurs when not sick
   b. is not due to effects of some medication

Encopresis

1. has had bowel movement outside of toilet after kindergarten
2. happens when not sick

Schizophrenia/Psychosis

A: Psychotic Symptoms

1. a. feels someone is out to harm him/her
   b. feels someone is trying to make him/her sick
   c. people seem to be against him/her
   d. people seem to talk about him/her
   e. people spy on him/her
2. a. eyes play tricks on him/her
   b. during daylight
   c. only when falling asleep
   d. ears play tricks on him/her
   e. voices talk about child's feelings/thoughts/acts
   f. voices talk to each other

Interviewer observed:
3. *incoherent speech*
4. *disorganized or catatonic behavior*
5. *inappropriate affect or inability to speak*

B: Interference

1. since problems started, has more difficulty getting along with other people
2. since problems started, does worse in school
3. since problems started, is careless about looks/hygiene

Psychosocial Stressors

A: Child Abuse/Neglect

1. a. M/F criticizes child a lot
   b. M/F wishes child had never been born
   c. M/F says he/she hates child
2. a. M/F ignores child
   b. M/F misses child's doctor appointments
   c. M/F does not feed child
   d. M/F does not clothe child
3. a. child is spanked or hit
   b. child is sometimes spanked or hit for no reason
   c. child fears physical harm from M/F
   d. child has been bruised, sore, taken to doctor
4. child has been sexually abused
5. child has been made to go a whole day without food

B: Other Stressors

1. a. fighting within family
   b. among children
   c. between parents
   d. between parents and children
   e. fighting bothers child
2. child remembers parents' separation/divorce
3. a. family has money problems
   b. child is worried about money problems
4. a. family member is ill
   b. family member has been hospitalized
   c. child worries
5. a. family member drinks or uses drugs a lot
   b. child worries
6. a. family member has been in trouble with police
   b. child worries
7. a. someone close to child has gotten sick and died
   b. child was very upset
8. a. someone close to child was murdered
   b. child was very upset
   c. someone close to child was killed in an accident
   d. child was very upset
9. anything else we need to know so we can help you?
   _____
   _____
10. problems child thinks he/she needs help with?
   _____
   _____
11. anything in the interview that bothered you?
   _____
   _____

P-ChIPS Report Form

Child's Name: _____ Date: _____ / _____ / _____

Informant's Name: _____ Interviewer: _____

Informant's Relationship (circle one): Mother, Father, Stepmother, Stepfather, Guardian, Other _____

Attention-Deficit/Hyperactivity Disorder

A: Inattention
1. a. pays no attention to details
   b. makes careless mistakes on schoolwork
2. can't keep mind on what he/she is doing
3. a. has trouble listening to parent
   b. has trouble listening to teacher
4. has trouble finishing things
5. has trouble organizing self
6. avoids schoolwork
7. loses school supplies
8. a. is easily distracted
   b. teacher reports inattention/daydreaming
9. a. is forgetful
   b. teacher reports forgetfulness

B: Hyperactivity–Impulsivity
1. a. is often told to sit still
   b. is constantly moving hands/feet
2. a. has trouble staying in seat
   b. gets in trouble for getting out of chair
3. gets in trouble for running/climbing
4. a. is too loud when playing
   b. has difficulty playing quietly
5. teacher reports is always "on the go"
6. a. talks out of turn at school
   b. talks too much at home
7. blurts out answers to questions
8. a. pushes ahead in line
   b. can't wait for his/her turn in games
9. a. barges in on other kids' games
   b. pushes into others' groups
   c. interrupts busy people

Oppositional Defiant Disorder
1. a. loses temper when things don't go his/her way
   b. has frequent temper tantrums
2. a. talks back/argues with parents
   b. talks back/argues with teachers
3. a. breaks rules at home
   b. breaks rules at school
   c. refuses to follow teachers' directions
   d. disobeys direct orders
4. purposely "bugs" other people
5. blames others for his/her own mistakes
6. is easily angered by others
7. is angry a lot of the time
8. gets even when angered

Conduct Disorder
1. has stolen >1 time
2. a. lies to get out of doing things
   b. "cons" people
3. has broken into a car or building to steal
4. has skipped school >3 times
5. breaks curfew >1 time per month
6. has run away/stayed out all night >1 time *or* did not return for a long time
7. a. is a bully
   b. threatens other people
8. a. is avoided because he/she starts fights
   b. gets in trouble for fighting
9. has used a weapon in a fight >1 time
10. a. has hurt someone badly in a fight
    b. has hurt someone for no reason
11. has taken things from people by force
12. has damaged property
13. has set something on fire (>1 time *or* caused extensive damage)
14. has hurt or killed an animal for fun
15. a. has forcefully performed sexual activity on another
    b. has forced someone to perform sexual activity on him-/herself

Substance Abuse
1. a. has smoked cigarettes ≥2 times _____
   b. has smoked pot ≥2 times _____
   c. has smoked other drugs ≥2 times _____
2. has used alcohol _____
3. has used other drugs _____
4. has sniffed a substance ≥2 times _____

Specific Phobia

1. phobic object/situation: _____
2. when confronted with object/situation,
   a. gets uptight and scared, can't move
   b. cries, clings to parents, throws tantrums
3. a. avoids object/situation
   b. becomes nauseated, feels faint
4. a. fear interferes with (sleep, school, activities)
   b. feels *super* uncomfortable because of fear
5. a. is more scared of object/situation than peers
   b. fear seems silly to child

Social Phobia

1. a. is afraid of being around other people
   b. has fear of performing
2. feels super-uncomfortable when a/b occurs
3. a. tries to avoid social situations
   b. if unavoidable, feels awful
4. a. fear interferes with (sleep, school, activities)
   b. feels *super* uncomfortable because of fear
5. behavior seems silly to child

Separation Anxiety

1. a. cries, begs parent to stay home
   b. tries to stay home with parent at all times
2. a. worries about parent getting harmed
   b. fears parental harm if separated
3. fears personal harm when separated from parent
4. a. has difficulty going to school
   b. refuses to go to school
5. a. is afraid to be in room of house alone
   b. follows parent around the house
6. a. can't sleep if not with parent
   b. can't sleep away from home
7. a. has nightmares about separation
   b. has nightmares about parental loss
8. a. has stomach- or headaches before going to school
   b. gets ill when parent leaves him/her

Generalized Anxiety Disorder

1. worries more than other kids _____
2. a. has difficulty calming down
   b. can't let go of worry
3. when worried, feels edgy, tired, distractible, cranky; has tight muscles, poor sleep

Obsessive-Compulsive Disorder

A: Compulsions

1. does things over and over
2. a. feels behavior will improve things
   b. thinks that if he/she can't perform behavior, something bad will happen
3. feels that behavior does not make sense

B: Obsessions

1. a. has bothersome thoughts/ideas
   b. "sees" pictures in head repeatedly
   c. has to do something but never does it
2. a. tries to make bothersome thoughts go away
   b. tries to pretend that thoughts aren't there
   c. does other things to try to make thoughts go away

3. thoughts seem like child's own (as opposed to someone else putting thoughts in his/her mind)

C: Interference

1. a. thoughts/behaviors cause child discomfort
   b. thoughts/behaviors cause problems at (home, school, play)
   c. thoughts/behaviors interfere with daily routines (time spent daily: _____)

Stress Disorders—PTSD, ASD

A: Exposure

1. a. child experienced traumatic event _____
   b. child witnessed traumatic event happening to someone else _____
2. after event, felt helpless, shocked, horrified, like he/she was falling apart; was hard to calm down
3. how long ago did event happen? _____

B: Dissociation

1. after event, felt cut off from family/friends; felt fewer emotions, felt numb
2. felt out of touch, in a daze
3. felt that the world was not real
4. felt that self was no longer real
5. had trouble remembering event

C: Reexperiencing

1. a. replays event over and over in mind
   b. "sees" event happening again
   c. plays games about event over and over
2. a. has nightmares about event
   b. has nightmares but can't remember what they're about
3. a. "feels" event happening again
   b. acts like event is happening again
4. a. becomes upset when reminded of event
   b. becomes upset when in same physical setting in which event occurred
5. when reminded of event, gets anxious, achy, sweaty palms, breathing problems

D: Avoidance

1. a. avoids thinking/talking about event
   b. tries to be unafraid of anything
2. a. avoids activities that remind him/her of event
   b. avoids places that remind him/her of event
   c. avoids people that remind him/her of event
3. can't remember things about event
4. a. has decreased interest in things he/she used to enjoy
   b. has stopped doing things he/she used to enjoy
5. feels cut off from family/friends
6. feels fewer emotions; feels numb
7. a. feels he/she won't grow up
   b. feels he/she will die soon

E: Hyperarousal

1. a. has trouble falling asleep
   b. has trouble staying asleep
2. a. is harder to get along with
   b. is easily angered
3. has difficulty concentrating
4. is super-alert
5. is easily startled, jumpy

Anorexia

1. a. has lost weight by dieting
   b. tries to stay underweight
2. a. current weight and height _____
   b. weight and height when thinnest _____
3. a. is terrified of getting fat
   b. is afraid of gaining weight
   c. fears he/she won't stop eating if he/she starts
4. a. feels fat
   b. feels good/bad depending on weight
   c. thinks his/her weight is a problem
5. if she's started menstruation yet, amenorrhea?

Bulimia

1. eats lots of food in short time
2. feels he/she can't stop eating, only stops because

   _____
3. after eating, tries to lose weight by . . .
   a. not eating
   b. vomiting
   c. taking laxatives
   d. overexercising
4. a. is more weight-conscious than peers
   b. self-image depends on weight

Depression/Dysthymia

A: Dysphoric Mood
1. a. feels sad or depressed
   b. almost every day
   c. lasts most of the day
2. a. feels more irritable
   b. (i) fights (ii) cries (iii) temper
   c. almost every day
   d. lasts most of the day

B: Loss of Interest
1. a. used to have fun doing _____
   b. isn't fun anymore
2. a. wants to have fun but can't
   b. feels that nothing is fun anymore
   c. has lost interest in daily activities

C: Appetite Changes
1. a. has decreased appetite
   b. has lost weight without dieting
   c. clothes are too big now
2. a. has increased appetite
   b. has gained weight

D: Sleep Changes
1. goes to bed @ _____; wakes @ _____
   a. early insomnia
   b. middle insomnia
   c. late insomnia
2. a. naps a lot
   b. hypersomnia

E: Psychomotor Changes
1. a. can't sit still
   b. is fidgety
   c. wrings hands
   d. picks at him-/herself
2. a. takes longer to do things
   b. has difficulty doing anything

F: Low Energy
1. a. has no energy
   b. has to push self
   c. tires easily
   d. sits around, does nothing

G: Guilt
1. a. has bad thoughts about self
   b. feels down on self
   c. feels he/she is no good
   d. hates self
2. a. feels guilty a lot
   b. thinks he/she should be punished

H: Impaired Concentration
1. a. mind has slowed down
   b. forgets things more
   c. has trouble paying attention
   d. listens to teacher less than before
   e. grades have dropped
2. has difficulty making up mind

I: Hopelessness
1. a. feels that nothing good will happen in the future
   b. feels that things won't get any better
   c. feels that there's no hope for the future

J: Morbid/Suicidal Thoughts
1. a. thinks about death
   b. thinks about dead people/pets
2. a. wishes he/she were dead
   b. feels life isn't worth living
   c. has thought of suicide
   d. has thought of suicide plans
   e. has made suicide attempt

Mania/Hypomania

A: Elevated Mood
1. a. feels very, very good
   b. feels wonderful for no reason
   c. is "too high"
2. has discrete periods of irritability

B: Other Symptoms
1. a. believes he/she has special abilities
   b. believes he/she can do things better than anyone
2. a. has lots of energy, no need for sleep
   b. sleeps a lot less without feeling tired
   c. needs ≤3 hours of sleep to feel OK
3. a. has rapid, unstoppable speech
   b. talks so fast that family/friends worry
   c. is told he/she talks too much, too loudly
   d. talks too fast to be understood
4. a. thoughts race through mind
   b. thoughts come too fast to verbalize them all
   c. feels that mind is sped up, working too fast
5. has trouble focusing
6. a. does more things than usual
   b. has more energy than usual
   c. tries many different things
   d. family/friends are concerned
   e. is more active than usual
7. a. gets in trouble more
   b. does things he/she usually wouldn't
   c. gets hurt due to carelessness
   d. is a lot more interested in sex than usual

C: Interference
1. mood/behavior causes problems at (home, school, play)
2. mood/behavior is reason child is here

Enuresis

1. has wet bed after kindergarten
2. a. wets bed at night
   b. wets self during day
3. a. occurs when not sick
   b. is not due to effects of some medication

Encopresis

1. has had bowel movement outside of toilet after kindergarten
2. happens when not sick

Schizophrenia/Psychosis

A: Psychotic Symptoms

1. a. feels someone is out to harm him/her
   b. feels someone is trying to make him/her sick
   c. people seem to be against him/her
   d. people seem to talk about him/her
   e. people spy on him/her
2. a. eyes play tricks on him/her
   b. during daylight
   c. only when falling asleep
   d. ears play tricks on him/her
   e. voices talk about child's feelings/thoughts/acts
   f. voices talk to each other

Interviewer observed:
3. *incoherent speech*
4. *disorganized or catatonic behavior*
5. *inappropriate affect or inability to speak*

B: Interference

1. since problems started, has more difficulty getting along with other people
2. since problems started, does worse in school
3. since problems started, is careless about looks/hygiene

Psychosocial Stressors

A: Child Abuse/Neglect

1. a. M/F criticizes child a lot
   b. M/F wishes child had never been born
   c. M/F says he/she hates child
2. a. M/F ignores child
   b. M/F misses child's doctor appointments
   c. M/F does not feed child
   d. M/F does not clothe child
3. a. child is spanked or hit
   b. child is sometimes spanked or hit for no reason
   c. child fears physical harm from M/F
   d. child has been bruised, sore, taken to doctor
4. child has been sexually abused
5. child has been made to go a whole day without food

B: Other Stressors

1. a. fighting within family
   b. among children
   c. between parents
   d. between parents and children
   e. fighting bothers child
2. child remembers parents' separation/divorce
3. a. family has money problems
   b. child is worried about money problems
4. a. family member is ill
   b. family member has been hospitalized
   c. child worries
5. a. family member drinks or uses drugs a lot
   b. child worries
6. a. family member has been in trouble with police
   b. child worries
7. a. someone close to child has gotten sick and died
   b. child was very upset
8. a. someone close to child was murdered
   b. child was very upset
   c. someone close to child was killed in an accident
   d. child was very upset
9. anything else we need to know so we can help you?
   _____
   _____
10. problems child thinks he/she needs help with?
    _____
    _____
11. anything in the interview that bothered you?
    _____
    _____

P-ChIPS Report Form

Child's Name: _____ Date: ____ / _____ / _____

Informant's Name: _____ Interviewer: _____

Informant's Relationship (circle one): Mother, Father, Stepmother, Stepfather, Guardian, Other _____

Attention-Deficit/Hyperactivity Disorder

A: Inattention

1. a. pays no attention to details
   b. makes careless mistakes on schoolwork
2. can't keep mind on what he/she is doing
3. a. has trouble listening to parent
   b. has trouble listening to teacher
4. has trouble finishing things
5. has trouble organizing self
6. avoids schoolwork
7. loses school supplies
8. a. is easily distracted
   b. teacher reports inattention/daydreaming
9. a. is forgetful
   b. teacher reports forgetfulness

B: Hyperactivity–Impulsivity

1. a. is often told to sit still
   b. is constantly moving hands/feet
2. a. has trouble staying in seat
   b. gets in trouble for getting out of chair
3. gets in trouble for running/climbing
4. a. is too loud when playing
   b. has difficulty playing quietly
5. teacher reports is always "on the go"
6. a. talks out of turn at school
   b. talks too much at home
7. blurts out answers to questions
8. a. pushes ahead in line
   b. can't wait for his/her turn in games
9. a. barges in on other kids' games
   b. pushes into others' groups
   c. interrupts busy people

Oppositional Defiant Disorder

1. a. loses temper when things don't go his/her way
   b. has frequent temper tantrums
2. a. talks back/argues with parents
   b. talks back/argues with teachers
3. a. breaks rules at home
   b. breaks rules at school
   c. refuses to follow teachers' directions
   d. disobeys direct orders
4. purposely "bugs" other people
5. blames others for his/her own mistakes
6. is easily angered by others
7. is angry a lot of the time
8. gets even when angered

Conduct Disorder

1. has stolen >1 time
2. a. lies to get out of doing things
   b. "cons" people
3. has broken into a car or building to steal
4. has skipped school >3 times
5. breaks curfew >1 time per month
6. has run away/stayed out all night >1 time *or* did not return for a long time
7. a. is a bully
   b. threatens other people
8. a. is avoided because he/she starts fights
   b. gets in trouble for fighting
9. has used a weapon in a fight >1 time
10. a. has hurt someone badly in a fight
    b. has hurt someone for no reason
11. has taken things from people by force
12. has damaged property
13. has set something on fire (>1 time *or* caused extensive damage)
14. has hurt or killed an animal for fun
15. a. has forcefully performed sexual activity on another
    b. has forced someone to perform sexual activity on him-/herself

Substance Abuse

1. a. has smoked cigarettes ≥2 times _____
   b. has smoked pot ≥2 times _____
   c. has smoked other drugs ≥2 times _____
2. has used alcohol _____
3. has used other drugs _____
4. has sniffed a substance ≥2 times _____

Specific Phobia

1. phobic object/situation: _____
2. when confronted with object/situation,
   a. gets uptight and scared, can't move
   b. cries, clings to parents, throws tantrums
3. a. avoids object/situation
   b. becomes nauseated, feels faint
4. a. fear interferes with (sleep, school, activities)
   b. feels *super* uncomfortable because of fear
5. a. is more scared of object/situation than peers
   b. fear seems silly to child

Social Phobia

1. a. is afraid of being around other people
   b. has fear of performing
2. feels super-uncomfortable when a/b occurs
3. a. tries to avoid social situations
   b. if unavoidable, feels awful
4. a. fear interferes with (sleep, school, activities)
   b. feels *super* uncomfortable because of fear
5. behavior seems silly to child

Separation Anxiety

1. a. cries, begs parent to stay home
   b. tries to stay home with parent at all times
2. a. worries about parent getting harmed
   b. fears parental harm if separated
3. fears personal harm when separated from parent
4. a. has difficulty going to school
   b. refuses to go to school
5. a. is afraid to be in room of house alone
   b. follows parent around the house
6. a. can't sleep if not with parent
   b. can't sleep away from home
7. a. has nightmares about separation
   b. has nightmares about parental loss
8. a. has stomach- or headaches before going to school
   b. gets ill when parent leaves him/her

Generalized Anxiety Disorder

1. worries more than other kids _____
2. a. has difficulty calming down
   b. can't let go of worry
3. when worried, feels edgy, tired, distractible, cranky; has tight muscles, poor sleep

Obsessive-Compulsive Disorder

A: Compulsions

1. does things over and over
2. a. feels behavior will improve things
   b. thinks that if he/she can't perform behavior, something bad will happen
3. feels that behavior does not make sense

B: Obsessions

1. a. has bothersome thoughts/ideas
   b. "sees" pictures in head repeatedly
   c. has to do something but never does it
2. a. tries to make bothersome thoughts go away
   b. tries to pretend that thoughts aren't there
   c. does other things to try to make thoughts go away

3. thoughts seem like child's own (as opposed to someone else putting thoughts in his/her mind)

C: Interference

1. a. thoughts/behaviors cause child discomfort
   b. thoughts/behaviors cause problems at (home, school, play)
   c. thoughts/behaviors interfere with daily routines (time spent daily: _____)

Stress Disorders—PTSD, ASD

A: Exposure

1. a. child experienced traumatic event _____
   b. child witnessed traumatic event happening to someone else _____
2. after event, felt helpless, shocked, horrified, like he/she was falling apart; was hard to calm down
3. how long ago did event happen? _____

B: Dissociation

1. after event, felt cut off from family/friends; felt fewer emotions, felt numb
2. felt out of touch, in a daze
3. felt that the world was not real
4. felt that self was no longer real
5. had trouble remembering event

C: Reexperiencing

1. a. replays event over and over in mind
   b. "sees" event happening again
   c. plays games about event over and over
2. a. has nightmares about event
   b. has nightmares but can't remember what they're about
3. a. "feels" event happening again
   b. acts like event is happening again
4. a. becomes upset when reminded of event
   b. becomes upset when in same physical setting in which event occurred
5. when reminded of event, gets anxious, achy, sweaty palms, breathing problems

D: Avoidance

1. a. avoids thinking/talking about event
   b. tries to be unafraid of anything
2. a. avoids activities that remind him/her of event
   b. avoids places that remind him/her of event
   c. avoids people that remind him/her of event
3. can't remember things about event
4. a. has decreased interest in things he/she used to enjoy
   b. has stopped doing things he/she used to enjoy
5. feels cut off from family/friends
6. feels fewer emotions; feels numb
7. a. feels he/she won't grow up
   b. feels he/she will die soon

E: Hyperarousal

1. a. has trouble falling asleep
   b. has trouble staying asleep
2. a. is harder to get along with
   b. is easily angered
3. has difficulty concentrating
4. is super-alert
5. is easily startled, jumpy

Anorexia

1. a. has lost weight by dieting
   b. tries to stay underweight
2. a. current weight and height _____
   b. weight and height when thinnest _____
3. a. is terrified of getting fat
   b. is afraid of gaining weight
   c. fears he/she won't stop eating if he/she starts
4. a. feels fat
   b. feels good/bad depending on weight
   c. thinks his/her weight is a problem
5. if she's started menstruation yet, amenorrhea?

Bulimia

1. eats lots of food in short time
2. feels he/she can't stop eating, only stops because
   _____
3. after eating, tries to lose weight by . . .
   a. not eating
   b. vomiting
   c. taking laxatives
   d. overexercising
4. a. is more weight-conscious than peers
   b. self-image depends on weight

Depression/Dysthymia

A: Dysphoric Mood
1. a. feels sad or depressed
   b. almost every day
   c. lasts most of the day
2. a. feels more irritable
   b. (i) fights (ii) cries (iii) temper
   c. almost every day
   d. lasts most of the day

B: Loss of Interest
1. a. used to have fun doing _____
   b. isn't fun anymore
2. a. wants to have fun but can't
   b. feels that nothing is fun anymore
   c. has lost interest in daily activities

C: Appetite Changes
1. a. has decreased appetite
   b. has lost weight without dieting
   c. clothes are too big now
2. a. has increased appetite
   b. has gained weight

D: Sleep Changes
1. goes to bed @ _____; wakes @ _____
   a. early insomnia
   b. middle insomnia
   c. late insomnia
2. a. naps a lot
   b. hypersomnia

E: Psychomotor Changes
1. a. can't sit still
   b. is fidgety
   c. wrings hands
   d. picks at him-/herself
2. a. takes longer to do things
   b. has difficulty doing anything

F: Low Energy
1. a. has no energy
   b. has to push self
   c. tires easily
   d. sits around, does nothing

G: Guilt
1. a. has bad thoughts about self
   b. feels down on self
   c. feels he/she is no good
   d. hates self
2. a. feels guilty a lot
   b. thinks he/she should be punished

H: Impaired Concentration
1. a. mind has slowed down
   b. forgets things more
   c. has trouble paying attention
   d. listens to teacher less than before
   e. grades have dropped
2. has difficulty making up mind

I: Hopelessness
1. a. feels that nothing good will happen in the future
   b. feels that things won't get any better
   c. feels that there's no hope for the future

J: Morbid/Suicidal Thoughts
1. a. thinks about death
   b. thinks about dead people/pets
2. a. wishes he/she were dead
   b. feels life isn't worth living
   c. has thought of suicide
   d. has thought of suicide plans
   e. has made suicide attempt

Mania/Hypomania

A: Elevated Mood
1. a. feels very, very good
   b. feels wonderful for no reason
   c. is "too high"
2. has discrete periods of irritability

B: Other Symptoms
1. a. believes he/she has special abilities
   b. believes he/she can do things better than anyone
2. a. has lots of energy, no need for sleep
   b. sleeps a lot less without feeling tired
   c. needs ≤3 hours of sleep to feel OK
3. a. has rapid, unstoppable speech
   b. talks so fast that family/friends worry
   c. is told he/she talks too much, too loudly
   d. talks too fast to be understood
4. a. thoughts race through mind
   b. thoughts come too fast to verbalize them all
   c. feels that mind is sped up, working too fast
5. has trouble focusing
6. a. does more things than usual
   b. has more energy than usual
   c. tries many different things
   d. family/friends are concerned
   e. is more active than usual
7. a. gets in trouble more
   b. does things he/she usually wouldn't
   c. gets hurt due to carelessness
   d. is a lot more interested in sex than usual

C: Interference
1. mood/behavior causes problems at (home, school, play)
2. mood/behavior is reason child is here

Enuresis

1. has wet bed after kindergarten
2. a. wets bed at night
   b. wets self during day
3. a. occurs when not sick
   b. is not due to effects of some medication

Encopresis

1. has had bowel movement outside of toilet after kindergarten
2. happens when not sick

Schizophrenia/Psychosis

A: Psychotic Symptoms

1. a. feels someone is out to harm him/her
   b. feels someone is trying to make him/her sick
   c. people seem to be against him/her
   d. people seem to talk about him/her
   e. people spy on him/her
2. a. eyes play tricks on him/her
   b. during daylight
   c. only when falling asleep
   d. ears play tricks on him/her
   e. voices talk about child's feelings/thoughts/acts
   f. voices talk to each other

Interviewer observed:
3. *incoherent speech*
4. *disorganized or catatonic behavior*
5. *inappropriate affect or inability to speak*

B: Interference

1. since problems started, has more difficulty getting along with other people
2. since problems started, does worse in school
3. since problems started, is careless about looks/ hygiene

Psychosocial Stressors

A: Child Abuse/Neglect

1. a. M/F criticizes child a lot
   b. M/F wishes child had never been born
   c. M/F says he/she hates child
2. a. M/F ignores child
   b. M/F misses child's doctor appointments
   c. M/F does not feed child
   d. M/F does not clothe child
3. a. child is spanked or hit
   b. child is sometimes spanked or hit for no reason
   c. child fears physical harm from M/F
   d. child has been bruised, sore, taken to doctor
4. child has been sexually abused
5. child has been made to go a whole day without food

B: Other Stressors

1. a. fighting within family
   b. among children
   c. between parents
   d. between parents and children
   e. fighting bothers child
2. child remembers parents' separation/divorce
3. a. family has money problems
   b. child is worried about money problems
4. a. family member is ill
   b. family member has been hospitalized
   c. child worries
5. a. family member drinks or uses drugs a lot
   b. child worries
6. a. family member has been in trouble with police
   b. child worries
7. a. someone close to child has gotten sick and died
   b. child was very upset
8. a. someone close to child was murdered
   b. child was very upset
   c. someone close to child was killed in an accident
   d. child was very upset
9. anything else we need to know so we can help you?
   _____
   _____
10. problems child thinks he/she needs help with?
    _____
    _____
11. anything in the interview that bothered you?
    _____
    _____

P-ChIPS Report Form

Child's Name: _____ Date: _____ / _____ / _____

Informant's Name: _____ Interviewer: _____

Informant's Relationship (circle one): Mother, Father, Stepmother, Stepfather, Guardian, Other _____

Attention-Deficit/Hyperactivity Disorder

A: Inattention

1. a. pays no attention to details
   b. makes careless mistakes on schoolwork
2. can't keep mind on what he/she is doing
3. a. has trouble listening to parent
   b. has trouble listening to teacher
4. has trouble finishing things
5. has trouble organizing self
6. avoids schoolwork
7. loses school supplies
8. a. is easily distracted
   b. teacher reports inattention/daydreaming
9. a. is forgetful
   b. teacher reports forgetfulness

B: Hyperactivity–Impulsivity

1. a. is often told to sit still
   b. is constantly moving hands/feet
2. a. has trouble staying in seat
   b. gets in trouble for getting out of chair
3. gets in trouble for running/climbing
4. a. is too loud when playing
   b. has difficulty playing quietly
5. teacher reports is always "on the go"
6. a. talks out of turn at school
   b. talks too much at home
7. blurts out answers to questions
8. a. pushes ahead in line
   b. can't wait for his/her turn in games
9. a. barges in on other kids' games
   b. pushes into others' groups
   c. interrupts busy people

Oppositional Defiant Disorder

1. a. loses temper when things don't go his/her way
   b. has frequent temper tantrums
2. a. talks back/argues with parents
   b. talks back/argues with teachers
3. a. breaks rules at home
   b. breaks rules at school
   c. refuses to follow teachers' directions
   d. disobeys direct orders
4. purposely "bugs" other people
5. blames others for his/her own mistakes
6. is easily angered by others
7. is angry a lot of the time
8. gets even when angered

Conduct Disorder

1. has stolen >1 time
2. a. lies to get out of doing things
   b. "cons" people
3. has broken into a car or building to steal
4. has skipped school >3 times
5. breaks curfew >1 time per month
6. has run away/stayed out all night >1 time or did not return for a long time
7. a. is a bully
   b. threatens other people
8. a. is avoided because he/she starts fights
   b. gets in trouble for fighting
9. has used a weapon in a fight >1 time
10. a. has hurt someone badly in a fight
    b. has hurt someone for no reason
11. has taken things from people by force
12. has damaged property
13. has set something on fire (>1 time or caused extensive damage)
14. has hurt or killed an animal for fun
15. a. has forcefully performed sexual activity on another
    b. has forced someone to perform sexual activity on him-/herself

Substance Abuse

1. a. has smoked cigarettes ≥2 times _____
   b. has smoked pot ≥2 times _____
   c. has smoked other drugs ≥2 times _____
2. has used alcohol _____
3. has used other drugs _____
4. has sniffed a substance ≥2 times _____

Specific Phobia

1. phobic object/situation: _____
2. when confronted with object/situation,
   a. gets uptight and scared, can't move
   b. cries, clings to parents, throws tantrums
3. a. avoids object/situation
   b. becomes nauseated, feels faint
4. a. fear interferes with (sleep, school, activities)
   b. feels *super* uncomfortable because of fear
5. a. is more scared of object/situation than peers
   b. fear seems silly to child

Social Phobia

1. a. is afraid of being around other people
   b. has fear of performing
2. feels super-uncomfortable when a/b occurs
3. a. tries to avoid social situations
   b. if unavoidable, feels awful
4. a. fear interferes with (sleep, school, activities)
   b. feels *super* uncomfortable because of fear
5. behavior seems silly to child

Separation Anxiety

1. a. cries, begs parent to stay home
   b. tries to stay home with parent at all times
2. a. worries about parent getting harmed
   b. fears parental harm if separated
3. fears personal harm when separated from parent
4. a. has difficulty going to school
   b. refuses to go to school
5. a. is afraid to be in room of house alone
   b. follows parent around the house
6. a. can't sleep if not with parent
   b. can't sleep away from home
7. a. has nightmares about separation
   b. has nightmares about parental loss
8. a. has stomach- or headaches before going to school
   b. gets ill when parent leaves him/her

Generalized Anxiety Disorder

1. worries more than other kids _____
2. a. has difficulty calming down
   b. can't let go of worry
3. when worried, feels edgy, tired, distractible, cranky; has tight muscles, poor sleep

Obsessive-Compulsive Disorder

A: Compulsions

1. does things over and over
2. a. feels behavior will improve things
   b. thinks that if he/she can't perform behavior, something bad will happen
3. feels that behavior does not make sense

B: Obsessions

1. a. has bothersome thoughts/ideas
   b. "sees" pictures in head repeatedly
   c. has to do something but never does it
2. a. tries to make bothersome thoughts go away
   b. tries to pretend that thoughts aren't there
   c. does other things to try to make thoughts go away

3. thoughts seem like child's own (as opposed to someone else putting thoughts in his/her mind)

C: Interference

1. a. thoughts/behaviors cause child discomfort
   b. thoughts/behaviors cause problems at (home, school, play)
   c. thoughts/behaviors interfere with daily routines (time spent daily: _____)

Stress Disorders—PTSD, ASD

A: Exposure

1. a. child experienced traumatic event _____
   b. child witnessed traumatic event happening to someone else _____
2. after event, felt helpless, shocked, horrified, like he/she was falling apart; was hard to calm down
3. how long ago did event happen? _____

B: Dissociation

1. after event, felt cut off from family/friends; felt fewer emotions, felt numb
2. felt out of touch, in a daze
3. felt that the world was not real
4. felt that self was no longer real
5. had trouble remembering event

C: Reexperiencing

1. a. replays event over and over in mind
   b. "sees" event happening again
   c. plays games about event over and over
2. a. has nightmares about event
   b. has nightmares but can't remember what they're about
3. a. "feels" event happening again
   b. acts like event is happening again
4. a. becomes upset when reminded of event
   b. becomes upset when in same physical setting in which event occurred
5. when reminded of event, gets anxious, achy, sweaty palms, breathing problems

D: Avoidance

1. a. avoids thinking/talking about event
   b. tries to be unafraid of anything
2. a. avoids activities that remind him/her of event
   b. avoids places that remind him/her of event
   c. avoids people that remind him/her of event
3. can't remember things about event
4. a. has decreased interest in things he/she used to enjoy
   b. has stopped doing things he/she used to enjoy
5. feels cut off from family/friends
6. feels fewer emotions; feels numb
7. a. feels he/she won't grow up
   b. feels he/she will die soon

E: Hyperarousal

1. a. has trouble falling asleep
   b. has trouble staying asleep
2. a. is harder to get along with
   b. is easily angered
3. has difficulty concentrating
4. is super-alert
5. is easily startled, jumpy

Anorexia

1. a. has lost weight by dieting
   b. tries to stay underweight
2. a. current weight and height _____
   b. weight and height when thinnest _____
3. a. is terrified of getting fat
   b. is afraid of gaining weight
   c. fears he/she won't stop eating if he/she starts
4. a. feels fat
   b. feels good/bad depending on weight
   c. thinks his/her weight is a problem
5. if she's started menstruation yet, amenorrhea?

Bulimia

1. eats lots of food in short time
2. feels he/she can't stop eating, only stops because
   _____
3. after eating, tries to lose weight by . . .
   a. not eating
   b. vomiting
   c. taking laxatives
   d. overexercising
4. a. is more weight-conscious than peers
   b. self-image depends on weight

Depression/Dysthymia

A: Dysphoric Mood
1. a. feels sad or depressed
   b. almost every day
   c. lasts most of the day
2. a. feels more irritable
   b. (i) fights (ii) cries (iii) temper
   c. almost every day
   d. lasts most of the day

B: Loss of Interest
1. a. used to have fun doing _____
   b. isn't fun anymore
2. a. wants to have fun but can't
   b. feels that nothing is fun anymore
   c. has lost interest in daily activities

C: Appetite Changes
1. a. has decreased appetite
   b. has lost weight without dieting
   c. clothes are too big now
2. a. has increased appetite
   b. has gained weight

D: Sleep Changes
1. goes to bed @ _____; wakes @ _____
   a. early insomnia
   b. middle insomnia
   c. late insomnia
2. a. naps a lot
   b. hypersomnia

E: Psychomotor Changes
1. a. can't sit still
   b. is fidgety
   c. wrings hands
   d. picks at him-/herself
2. a. takes longer to do things
   b. has difficulty doing anything

F: Low Energy
1. a. has no energy
   b. has to push self
   c. tires easily
   d. sits around, does nothing

G: Guilt
1. a. has bad thoughts about self
   b. feels down on self
   c. feels he/she is no good
   d. hates self
2. a. feels guilty a lot
   b. thinks he/she should be punished

H: Impaired Concentration
1. a. mind has slowed down
   b. forgets things more
   c. has trouble paying attention
   d. listens to teacher less than before
   e. grades have dropped
2. has difficulty making up mind

I: Hopelessness
1. a. feels that nothing good will happen in the future
   b. feels that things won't get any better
   c. feels that there's no hope for the future

J: Morbid/Suicidal Thoughts
1. a. thinks about death
   b. thinks about dead people/pets
2. a. wishes he/she were dead
   b. feels life isn't worth living
   c. has thought of suicide
   d. has thought of suicide plans
   e. has made suicide attempt

Mania/Hypomania

A: Elevated Mood
1. a. feels very, very good
   b. feels wonderful for no reason
   c. is "too high"
2. has discrete periods of irritability

B: Other Symptoms
1. a. believes he/she has special abilities
   b. believes he/she can do things better than anyone
2. a. has lots of energy, no need for sleep
   b. sleeps a lot less without feeling tired
   c. needs ≤3 hours of sleep to feel OK
3. a. has rapid, unstoppable speech
   b. talks so fast that family/friends worry
   c. is told he/she talks too much, too loudly
   d. talks too fast to be understood
4. a. thoughts race through mind
   b. thoughts come too fast to verbalize them all
   c. feels that mind is sped up, working too fast
5. has trouble focusing
6. a. does more things than usual
   b. has more energy than usual
   c. tries many different things
   d. family/friends are concerned
   e. is more active than usual
7. a. gets in trouble more
   b. does things he/she usually wouldn't
   c. gets hurt due to carelessness
   d. is a lot more interested in sex than usual

C: Interference
1. mood/behavior causes problems at (home, school, play)
2. mood/behavior is reason child is here

Enuresis

1. has wet bed after kindergarten
2. a. wets bed at night
   b. wets self during day
3. a. occurs when not sick
   b. is not due to effects of some medication

Encopresis

1. has had bowel movement outside of toilet after kindergarten
2. happens when not sick

Schizophrenia/Psychosis

A: Psychotic Symptoms

1. a. feels someone is out to harm him/her
   b. feels someone is trying to make him/her sick
   c. people seem to be against him/her
   d. people seem to talk about him/her
   e. people spy on him/her
2. a. eyes play tricks on him/her
   b. during daylight
   c. only when falling asleep
   d. ears play tricks on him/her
   e. voices talk about child's feelings/thoughts/acts
   f. voices talk to each other

> *Interviewer observed:*
> 3. *incoherent speech*
> 4. *disorganized or catatonic behavior*
> 5. *inappropriate affect or inability to speak*

B: Interference

1. since problems started, has more difficulty getting along with other people
2. since problems started, does worse in school
3. since problems started, is careless about looks/hygiene

Psychosocial Stressors

A: Child Abuse/Neglect

1. a. M/F criticizes child a lot
   b. M/F wishes child had never been born
   c. M/F says he/she hates child
2. a. M/F ignores child
   b. M/F misses child's doctor appointments
   c. M/F does not feed child
   d. M/F does not clothe child
3. a. child is spanked or hit
   b. child is sometimes spanked or hit for no reason
   c. child fears physical harm from M/F
   d. child has been bruised, sore, taken to doctor
4. child has been sexually abused
5. child has been made to go a whole day without food

B: Other Stressors

1. a. fighting within family
   b. among children
   c. between parents
   d. between parents and children
   e. fighting bothers child
2. child remembers parents' separation/divorce
3. a. family has money problems
   b. child is worried about money problems
4. a. family member is ill
   b. family member has been hospitalized
   c. child worries
5. a. family member drinks or uses drugs a lot
   b. child worries
6. a. family member has been in trouble with police
   b. child worries
7. a. someone close to child has gotten sick and died
   b. child was very upset
8. a. someone close to child was murdered
   b. child was very upset
   c. someone close to child was killed in an accident
   d. child was very upset
9. anything else we need to know so we can help you?
   _____
   _____
10. problems child thinks he/she needs help with?
    _____
    _____
11. anything in the interview that bothered you?
    _____
    _____

P-ChIPS Report Form

Child's Name: _____ Date: ____ / _____ / _____

Informant's Name: _____ Interviewer: _____

Informant's Relationship (circle one): Mother, Father, Stepmother, Stepfather, Guardian, Other _____

Attention-Deficit/Hyperactivity Disorder

A: Inattention
1. a. pays no attention to details
   b. makes careless mistakes on schoolwork
2. can't keep mind on what he/she is doing
3. a. has trouble listening to parent
   b. has trouble listening to teacher
4. has trouble finishing things
5. has trouble organizing self
6. avoids schoolwork
7. loses school supplies
8. a. is easily distracted
   b. teacher reports inattention/daydreaming
9. a. is forgetful
   b. teacher reports forgetfulness

B: Hyperactivity–Impulsivity
1. a. is often told to sit still
   b. is constantly moving hands/feet
2. a. has trouble staying in seat
   b. gets in trouble for getting out of chair
3. gets in trouble for running/climbing
4. a. is too loud when playing
   b. has difficulty playing quietly
5. teacher reports is always "on the go"
6. a. talks out of turn at school
   b. talks too much at home
7. blurts out answers to questions
8. a. pushes ahead in line
   b. can't wait for his/her turn in games
9. a. barges in on other kids' games
   b. pushes into others' groups
   c. interrupts busy people

Oppositional Defiant Disorder
1. a. loses temper when things don't go his/her way
   b. has frequent temper tantrums
2. a. talks back/argues with parents
   b. talks back/argues with teachers
3. a. breaks rules at home
   b. breaks rules at school
   c. refuses to follow teachers' directions
   d. disobeys direct orders
4. purposely "bugs" other people
5. blames others for his/her own mistakes
6. is easily angered by others
7. is angry a lot of the time
8. gets even when angered

Conduct Disorder
1. has stolen >1 time
2. a. lies to get out of doing things
   b. "cons" people
3. has broken into a car or building to steal
4. has skipped school >3 times
5. breaks curfew >1 time per month
6. has run away/stayed out all night >1 time or did not return for a long time
7. a. is a bully
   b. threatens other people
8. a. is avoided because he/she starts fights
   b. gets in trouble for fighting
9. has used a weapon in a fight >1 time
10. a. has hurt someone badly in a fight
    b. has hurt someone for no reason
11. has taken things from people by force
12. has damaged property
13. has set something on fire (>1 time or caused extensive damage)
14. has hurt or killed an animal for fun
15. a. has forcefully performed sexual activity on another
    b. has forced someone to perform sexual activity on him-/herself

Substance Abuse
1. a. has smoked cigarettes ≥2 times _____
   b. has smoked pot ≥2 times _____
   c. has smoked other drugs ≥2 times _____
2. has used alcohol _____
3. has used other drugs _____
4. has sniffed a substance ≥2 times _____

Specific Phobia

1. phobic object/situation: _____
2. when confronted with object/situation,
   a. gets uptight and scared, can't move
   b. cries, clings to parents, throws tantrums
3. a. avoids object/situation
   b. becomes nauseated, feels faint
4. a. fear interferes with (sleep, school, activities)
   b. feels *super* uncomfortable because of fear
5. a. is more scared of object/situation than peers
   b. fear seems silly to child

Social Phobia

1. a. is afraid of being around other people
   b. has fear of performing
2. feels super-uncomfortable when a/b occurs
3. a. tries to avoid social situations
   b. if unavoidable, feels awful
4. a. fear interferes with (sleep, school, activities)
   b. feels *super* uncomfortable because of fear
5. behavior seems silly to child

Separation Anxiety

1. a. cries, begs parent to stay home
   b. tries to stay home with parent at all times
2. a. worries about parent getting harmed
   b. fears parental harm if separated
3. fears personal harm when separated from parent
4. a. has difficulty going to school
   b. refuses to go to school
5. a. is afraid to be in room of house alone
   b. follows parent around the house
6. a. can't sleep if not with parent
   b. can't sleep away from home
7. a. has nightmares about separation
   b. has nightmares about parental loss
8. a. has stomach- or headaches before going to school
   b. gets ill when parent leaves him/her

Generalized Anxiety Disorder

1. worries more than other kids _____
2. a. has difficulty calming down
   b. can't let go of worry
3. when worried, feels edgy, tired, distractible, cranky; has tight muscles, poor sleep

Obsessive-Compulsive Disorder

A: Compulsions

1. does things over and over
2. a. feels behavior will improve things
   b. thinks that if he/she can't perform behavior, something bad will happen
3. feels that behavior does not make sense

B: Obsessions

1. a. has bothersome thoughts/ideas
   b. "sees" pictures in head repeatedly
   c. has to do something but never does it
2. a. tries to make bothersome thoughts go away
   b. tries to pretend that thoughts aren't there
   c. does other things to try to make thoughts go away

3. thoughts seem like child's own (as opposed to someone else putting thoughts in his/her mind)

C: Interference

1. a. thoughts/behaviors cause child discomfort
   b. thoughts/behaviors cause problems at (home, school, play)
   c. thoughts/behaviors interfere with daily routines (time spent daily: _____)

Stress Disorders—PTSD, ASD

A: Exposure

1. a. child experienced traumatic event _____
   b. child witnessed traumatic event happening to someone else _____
2. after event, felt helpless, shocked, horrified, like he/she was falling apart; was hard to calm down
3. how long ago did event happen? _____

B: Dissociation

1. after event, felt cut off from family/friends; felt fewer emotions, felt numb
2. felt out of touch, in a daze
3. felt that the world was not real
4. felt that self was no longer real
5. had trouble remembering event

C: Reexperiencing

1. a. replays event over and over in mind
   b. "sees" event happening again
   c. plays games about event over and over
2. a. has nightmares about event
   b. has nightmares but can't remember what they're about
3. a. "feels" event happening again
   b. acts like event is happening again
4. a. becomes upset when reminded of event
   b. becomes upset when in same physical setting in which event occurred
5. when reminded of event, gets anxious, achy, sweaty palms, breathing problems

D: Avoidance

1. a. avoids thinking/talking about event
   b. tries to be unafraid of anything
2. a. avoids activities that remind him/her of event
   b. avoids places that remind him/her of event
   c. avoids people that remind him/her of event
3. can't remember things about event
4. a. has decreased interest in things he/she used to enjoy
   b. has stopped doing things he/she used to enjoy
5. feels cut off from family/friends
6. feels fewer emotions; feels numb
7. a. feels he/she won't grow up
   b. feels he/she will die soon

E: Hyperarousal

1. a. has trouble falling asleep
   b. has trouble staying asleep
2. a. is harder to get along with
   b. is easily angered
3. has difficulty concentrating
4. is super-alert
5. is easily startled, jumpy

Anorexia

1. a. has lost weight by dieting
   b. tries to stay underweight
2. a. current weight and height _____
   b. weight and height when thinnest _____
3. a. is terrified of getting fat
   b. is afraid of gaining weight
   c. fears he/she won't stop eating if he/she starts
4. a. feels fat
   b. feels good/bad depending on weight
   c. thinks his/her weight is a problem
5. if she's started menstruation yet, amenorrhea?

Bulimia

1. eats lots of food in short time
2. feels he/she can't stop eating, only stops because
   _____
3. after eating, tries to lose weight by . . .
   a. not eating
   b. vomiting
   c. taking laxatives
   d. overexercising
4. a. is more weight-conscious than peers
   b. self-image depends on weight

Depression/Dysthymia

A: Dysphoric Mood

1. a. feels sad or depressed
   b. almost every day
   c. lasts most of the day
2. a. feels more irritable
   b. (i) fights (ii) cries (iii) temper
   c. almost every day
   d. lasts most of the day

B: Loss of Interest

1. a. used to have fun doing _____
   b. isn't fun anymore
2. a. wants to have fun but can't
   b. feels that nothing is fun anymore
   c. has lost interest in daily activities

C: Appetite Changes

1. a. has decreased appetite
   b. has lost weight without dieting
   c. clothes are too big now
2. a. has increased appetite
   b. has gained weight

D: Sleep Changes

1. goes to bed @ _____; wakes @ _____
   a. early insomnia
   b. middle insomnia
   c. late insomnia
2. a. naps a lot
   b. hypersomnia

E: Psychomotor Changes

1. a. can't sit still
   b. is fidgety
   c. wrings hands
   d. picks at him-/herself
2. a. takes longer to do things
   b. has difficulty doing anything

F: Low Energy

1. a. has no energy
   b. has to push self
   c. tires easily
   d. sits around, does nothing

G: Guilt

1. a. has bad thoughts about self
   b. feels down on self
   c. feels he/she is no good
   d. hates self
2. a. feels guilty a lot
   b. thinks he/she should be punished

H: Impaired Concentration

1. a. mind has slowed down
   b. forgets things more
   c. has trouble paying attention
   d. listens to teacher less than before
   e. grades have dropped
2. has difficulty making up mind

I: Hopelessness

1. a. feels that nothing good will happen in the future
   b. feels that things won't get any better
   c. feels that there's no hope for the future

J: Morbid/Suicidal Thoughts

1. a. thinks about death
   b. thinks about dead people/pets
2. a. wishes he/she were dead
   b. feels life isn't worth living
   c. has thought of suicide
   d. has thought of suicide plans
   e. has made suicide attempt

Mania/Hypomania

A: Elevated Mood

1. a. feels very, very good
   b. feels wonderful for no reason
   c. is "too high"
2. has discrete periods of irritability

B: Other Symptoms

1. a. believes he/she has special abilities
   b. believes he/she can do things better than anyone
2. a. has lots of energy, no need for sleep
   b. sleeps a lot less without feeling tired
   c. needs ≤3 hours of sleep to feel OK
3. a. has rapid, unstoppable speech
   b. talks so fast that family/friends worry
   c. is told he/she talks too much, too loudly
   d. talks too fast to be understood
4. a. thoughts race through mind
   b. thoughts come too fast to verbalize them all
   c. feels that mind is sped up, working too fast
5. has trouble focusing
6. a. does more things than usual
   b. has more energy than usual
   c. tries many different things
   d. family/friends are concerned
   e. is more active than usual
7. a. gets in trouble more
   b. does things he/she usually wouldn't
   c. gets hurt due to carelessness
   d. is a lot more interested in sex than usual

C: Interference

1. mood/behavior causes problems at (home, school, play)
2. mood/behavior is reason child is here

Enuresis

1. has wet bed after kindergarten
2. a. wets bed at night
   b. wets self during day
3. a. occurs when not sick
   b. is not due to effects of some medication

Encopresis

1. has had bowel movement outside of toilet after kindergarten
2. happens when not sick

Schizophrenia/Psychosis

A: Psychotic Symptoms

1. a. feels someone is out to harm him/her
   b. feels someone is trying to make him/her sick
   c. people seem to be against him/her
   d. people seem to talk about him/her
   e. people spy on him/her
2. a. eyes play tricks on him/her
   b. during daylight
   c. only when falling asleep
   d. ears play tricks on him/her
   e. voices talk about child's feelings/thoughts/acts
   f. voices talk to each other

Interviewer observed:
3. *incoherent speech*
4. *disorganized or catatonic behavior*
5. *inappropriate affect or inability to speak*

B: Interference

1. since problems started, has more difficulty getting along with other people
2. since problems started, does worse in school
3. since problems started, is careless about looks/ hygiene

Psychosocial Stressors

A: Child Abuse/Neglect

1. a. M/F criticizes child a lot
   b. M/F wishes child had never been born
   c. M/F says he/she hates child
2. a. M/F ignores child
   b. M/F misses child's doctor appointments
   c. M/F does not feed child
   d. M/F does not clothe child
3. a. child is spanked or hit
   b. child is sometimes spanked or hit for no reason
   c. child fears physical harm from M/F
   d. child has been bruised, sore, taken to doctor
4. child has been sexually abused
5. child has been made to go a whole day without food

B: Other Stressors

1. a. fighting within family
   b. among children
   c. between parents
   d. between parents and children
   e. fighting bothers child
2. child remembers parents' separation/divorce
3. a. family has money problems
   b. child is worried about money problems
4. a. family member is ill
   b. family member has been hospitalized
   c. child worries
5. a. family member drinks or uses drugs a lot
   b. child worries
6. a. family member has been in trouble with police
   b. child worries
7. a. someone close to child has gotten sick and died
   b. child was very upset
8. a. someone close to child was murdered
   b. child was very upset
   c. someone close to child was killed in an accident
   d. child was very upset
9. anything else we need to know so we can help you?

   _____
   _____

10. problems child thinks he/she needs help with?

    _____
    _____

11. anything in the interview that bothered you?

    _____
    _____

P-ChIPS Report Form

Child's Name: _____ Date: _____ / _____ / _____

Informant's Name: _____ Interviewer: _____

Informant's Relationship (circle one): Mother, Father, Stepmother, Stepfather, Guardian, Other _____

Attention-Deficit/Hyperactivity Disorder

A: Inattention

1. a. pays no attention to details
   b. makes careless mistakes on schoolwork
2. can't keep mind on what he/she is doing
3. a. has trouble listening to parent
   b. has trouble listening to teacher
4. has trouble finishing things
5. has trouble organizing self
6. avoids schoolwork
7. loses school supplies
8. a. is easily distracted
   b. teacher reports inattention/daydreaming
9. a. is forgetful
   b. teacher reports forgetfulness

B: Hyperactivity–Impulsivity

1. a. is often told to sit still
   b. is constantly moving hands/feet
2. a. has trouble staying in seat
   b. gets in trouble for getting out of chair
3. gets in trouble for running/climbing
4. a. is too loud when playing
   b. has difficulty playing quietly
5. teacher reports is always "on the go"
6. a. talks out of turn at school
   b. talks too much at home
7. blurts out answers to questions
8. a. pushes ahead in line
   b. can't wait for his/her turn in games
9. a. barges in on other kids' games
   b. pushes into others' groups
   c. interrupts busy people

Oppositional Defiant Disorder

1. a. loses temper when things don't go his/her way
   b. has frequent temper tantrums
2. a. talks back/argues with parents
   b. talks back/argues with teachers
3. a. breaks rules at home
   b. breaks rules at school
   c. refuses to follow teachers' directions
   d. disobeys direct orders
4. purposely "bugs" other people
5. blames others for his/her own mistakes
6. is easily angered by others
7. is angry a lot of the time
8. gets even when angered

Conduct Disorder

1. has stolen >1 time
2. a. lies to get out of doing things
   b. "cons" people
3. has broken into a car or building to steal
4. has skipped school >3 times
5. breaks curfew >1 time per month
6. has run away/stayed out all night >1 time or did not return for a long time
7. a. is a bully
   b. threatens other people
8. a. is avoided because he/she starts fights
   b. gets in trouble for fighting
9. has used a weapon in a fight >1 time
10. a. has hurt someone badly in a fight
    b. has hurt someone for no reason
11. has taken things from people by force
12. has damaged property
13. has set something on fire (>1 time or caused extensive damage)
14. has hurt or killed an animal for fun
15. a. has forcefully performed sexual activity on another
    b. has forced someone to perform sexual activity on him-/herself

Substance Abuse

1. a. has smoked cigarettes ≥2 times _____
   b. has smoked pot ≥2 times _____
   c. has smoked other drugs ≥2 times _____
2. has used alcohol _____
3. has used other drugs _____
4. has sniffed a substance ≥2 times _____

Specific Phobia

1. phobic object/situation: _____
2. when confronted with object/situation,
    a. gets uptight and scared, can't move
    b. cries, clings to parents, throws tantrums
3. a. avoids object/situation
    b. becomes nauseated, feels faint
4. a. fear interferes with (sleep, school, activities)
    b. feels *super* uncomfortable because of fear
5. a. is more scared of object/situation than peers
    b. fear seems silly to child

Social Phobia

1. a. is afraid of being around other people
    b. has fear of performing
2. feels super-uncomfortable when a/b occurs
3. a. tries to avoid social situations
    b. if unavoidable, feels awful
4. a. fear interferes with (sleep, school, activities)
    b. feels *super* uncomfortable because of fear
5. behavior seems silly to child

Separation Anxiety

1. a. cries, begs parent to stay home
    b. tries to stay home with parent at all times
2. a. worries about parent getting harmed
    b. fears parental harm if separated
3. fears personal harm when separated from parent
4. a. has difficulty going to school
    b. refuses to go to school
5. a. is afraid to be in room of house alone
    b. follows parent around the house
6. a. can't sleep if not with parent
    b. can't sleep away from home
7. a. has nightmares about separation
    b. has nightmares about parental loss
8. a. has stomach- or headaches before going to school
    b. gets ill when parent leaves him/her

Generalized Anxiety Disorder

1. worries more than other kids _____
2. a. has difficulty calming down
    b. can't let go of worry
3. when worried, feels edgy, tired, distractible, cranky; has tight muscles, poor sleep

Obsessive-Compulsive Disorder

A: Compulsions

1. does things over and over
2. a. feels behavior will improve things
    b. thinks that if he/she can't perform behavior, something bad will happen
3. feels that behavior does not make sense

B: Obsessions

1. a. has bothersome thoughts/ideas
    b. "sees" pictures in head repeatedly
    c. has to do something but never does it
2. a. tries to make bothersome thoughts go away
    b. tries to pretend that thoughts aren't there
    c. does other things to try to make thoughts go away

3. thoughts seem like child's own (as opposed to someone else putting thoughts in his/her mind)

C: Interference

1. a. thoughts/behaviors cause child discomfort
    b. thoughts/behaviors cause problems at (home, school, play)
    c. thoughts/behaviors interfere with daily routines (time spent daily: _____)

Stress Disorders—PTSD, ASD

A: Exposure

1. a. child experienced traumatic event _____
    b. child witnessed traumatic event happening to someone else _____
2. after event, felt helpless, shocked, horrified, like he/she was falling apart; was hard to calm down
3. how long ago did event happen? _____

B: Dissociation

1. after event, felt cut off from family/friends; felt fewer emotions, felt numb
2. felt out of touch, in a daze
3. felt that the world was not real
4. felt that self was no longer real
5. had trouble remembering event

C: Reexperiencing

1. a. replays event over and over in mind
    b. "sees" event happening again
    c. plays games about event over and over
2. a. has nightmares about event
    b. has nightmares but can't remember what they're about
3. a. "feels" event happening again
    b. acts like event is happening again
4. a. becomes upset when reminded of event
    b. becomes upset when in same physical setting in which event occurred
5. when reminded of event, gets anxious, achy, sweaty palms, breathing problems

D: Avoidance

1. a. avoids thinking/talking about event
    b. tries to be unafraid of anything
2. a. avoids activities that remind him/her of event
    b. avoids places that remind him/her of event
    c. avoids people that remind him/her of event
3. can't remember things about event
4. a. has decreased interest in things he/she used to enjoy
    b. has stopped doing things he/she used to enjoy
5. feels cut off from family/friends
6. feels fewer emotions; feels numb
7. a. feels he/she won't grow up
    b. feels he/she will die soon

E: Hyperarousal

1. a. has trouble falling asleep
    b. has trouble staying asleep
2. a. is harder to get along with
    b. is easily angered
3. has difficulty concentrating
4. is super-alert
5. is easily startled, jumpy

Anorexia

1. a. has lost weight by dieting
   b. tries to stay underweight
2. a. current weight and height _____
   b. weight and height when thinnest _____
3. a. is terrified of getting fat
   b. is afraid of gaining weight
   c. fears he/she won't stop eating if he/she starts
4. a. feels fat
   b. feels good/bad depending on weight
   c. thinks his/her weight is a problem
5. if she's started menstruation yet, amenorrhea?

Bulimia

1. eats lots of food in short time
2. feels he/she can't stop eating, only stops because
   _____
3. after eating, tries to lose weight by . . .
   a. not eating
   b. vomiting
   c. taking laxatives
   d. overexercising
4. a. is more weight-conscious than peers
   b. self-image depends on weight

Depression/Dysthymia

A: Dysphoric Mood

1. a. feels sad or depressed
   b. almost every day
   c. lasts most of the day
2. a. feels more irritable
   b. (i) fights (ii) cries (iii) temper
   c. almost every day
   d. lasts most of the day

B: Loss of Interest

1. a. used to have fun doing _____
   b. isn't fun anymore
2. a. wants to have fun but can't
   b. feels that nothing is fun anymore
   c. has lost interest in daily activities

C: Appetite Changes

1. a. has decreased appetite
   b. has lost weight without dieting
   c. clothes are too big now
2. a. has increased appetite
   b. has gained weight

D: Sleep Changes

1. goes to bed @ _____; wakes @ _____
   a. early insomnia
   b. middle insomnia
   c. late insomnia
2. a. naps a lot
   b. hypersomnia

E: Psychomotor Changes

1. a. can't sit still
   b. is fidgety
   c. wrings hands
   d. picks at him-/herself
2. a. takes longer to do things
   b. has difficulty doing anything

F: Low Energy

1. a. has no energy
   b. has to push self
   c. tires easily
   d. sits around, does nothing

G: Guilt

1. a. has bad thoughts about self
   b. feels down on self
   c. feels he/she is no good
   d. hates self
2. a. feels guilty a lot
   b. thinks he/she should be punished

H: Impaired Concentration

1. a. mind has slowed down
   b. forgets things more
   c. has trouble paying attention
   d. listens to teacher less than before
   e. grades have dropped
2. has difficulty making up mind

I: Hopelessness

1. a. feels that nothing good will happen in the future
   b. feels that things won't get any better
   c. feels that there's no hope for the future

J: Morbid/Suicidal Thoughts

1. a. thinks about death
   b. thinks about dead people/pets
2. a. wishes he/she were dead
   b. feels life isn't worth living
   c. has thought of suicide
   d. has thought of suicide plans
   e. has made suicide attempt

Mania/Hypomania

A: Elevated Mood

1. a. feels very, very good
   b. feels wonderful for no reason
   c. is "too high"
2. has discrete periods of irritability

B: Other Symptoms

1. a. believes he/she has special abilities
   b. believes he/she can do things better than anyone
2. a. has lots of energy, no need for sleep
   b. sleeps a lot less without feeling tired
   c. needs ≤3 hours of sleep to feel OK
3. a. has rapid, unstoppable speech
   b. talks so fast that family/friends worry
   c. is told he/she talks too much, too loudly
   d. talks too fast to be understood
4. a. thoughts race through mind
   b. thoughts come too fast to verbalize them all
   c. feels that mind is sped up, working too fast
5. has trouble focusing
6. a. does more things than usual
   b. has more energy than usual
   c. tries many different things
   d. family/friends are concerned
   e. is more active than usual
7. a. gets in trouble more
   b. does things he/she usually wouldn't
   c. gets hurt due to carelessness
   d. is a lot more interested in sex than usual

C: Interference

1. mood/behavior causes problems at (home, school, play)
2. mood/behavior is reason child is here

Enuresis

1. has wet bed after kindergarten
2. a. wets bed at night
   b. wets self during day
3. a. occurs when not sick
   b. is not due to effects of some medication

Encopresis

1. has had bowel movement outside of toilet after kindergarten
2. happens when not sick

Schizophrenia/Psychosis

A: Psychotic Symptoms

1. a. feels someone is out to harm him/her
   b. feels someone is trying to make him/her sick
   c. people seem to be against him/her
   d. people seem to talk about him/her
   e. people spy on him/her
2. a. eyes play tricks on him/her
   b. during daylight
   c. only when falling asleep
   d. ears play tricks on him/her
   e. voices talk about child's feelings/thoughts/acts
   f. voices talk to each other

Interviewer observed:
3. *incoherent speech*
4. *disorganized or catatonic behavior*
5. *inappropriate affect or inability to speak*

B: Interference

1. since problems started, has more difficulty getting along with other people
2. since problems started, does worse in school
3. since problems started, is careless about looks/hygiene

Psychosocial Stressors

A: Child Abuse/Neglect

1. a. M/F criticizes child a lot
   b. M/F wishes child had never been born
   c. M/F says he/she hates child
2. a. M/F ignores child
   b. M/F misses child's doctor appointments
   c. M/F does not feed child
   d. M/F does not clothe child
3. a. child is spanked or hit
   b. child is sometimes spanked or hit for no reason
   c. child fears physical harm from M/F
   d. child has been bruised, sore, taken to doctor
4. child has been sexually abused
5. child has been made to go a whole day without food

B: Other Stressors

1. a. fighting within family
   b. among children
   c. between parents
   d. between parents and children
   e. fighting bothers child
2. child remembers parents' separation/divorce
3. a. family has money problems
   b. child is worried about money problems
4. a. family member is ill
   b. family member has been hospitalized
   c. child worries
5. a. family member drinks or uses drugs a lot
   b. child worries
6. a. family member has been in trouble with police
   b. child worries
7. a. someone close to child has gotten sick and died
   b. child was very upset
8. a. someone close to child was murdered
   b. child was very upset
   c. someone close to child was killed in an accident
   d. child was very upset
9. anything else we need to know so we can help you?
   _____
   _____
10. problems child thinks he/she needs help with?
   _____
   _____
11. anything in the interview that bothered you?
   _____
   _____

P-ChIPS Report Form

Child's Name: _____ Date: _____ / _____ / _____

Informant's Name: _____ Interviewer: _____

Informant's Relationship (circle one): Mother, Father, Stepmother, Stepfather, Guardian, Other _____

Attention-Deficit/Hyperactivity Disorder

A: Inattention

1. a. pays no attention to details
    b. makes careless mistakes on schoolwork
2. can't keep mind on what he/she is doing
3. a. has trouble listening to parent
    b. has trouble listening to teacher
4. has trouble finishing things
5. has trouble organizing self
6. avoids schoolwork
7. loses school supplies
8. a. is easily distracted
    b. teacher reports inattention/daydreaming
9. a. is forgetful
    b. teacher reports forgetfulness

B: Hyperactivity–Impulsivity

1. a. is often told to sit still
    b. is constantly moving hands/feet
2. a. has trouble staying in seat
    b. gets in trouble for getting out of chair
3. gets in trouble for running/climbing
4. a. is too loud when playing
    b. has difficulty playing quietly
5. teacher reports is always "on the go"
6. a. talks out of turn at school
    b. talks too much at home
7. blurts out answers to questions
8. a. pushes ahead in line
    b. can't wait for his/her turn in games
9. a. barges in on other kids' games
    b. pushes into others' groups
    c. interrupts busy people

Oppositional Defiant Disorder

1. a. loses temper when things don't go his/her way
    b. has frequent temper tantrums
2. a. talks back/argues with parents
    b. talks back/argues with teachers
3. a. breaks rules at home
    b. breaks rules at school
    c. refuses to follow teachers' directions
    d. disobeys direct orders
4. purposely "bugs" other people
5. blames others for his/her own mistakes
6. is easily angered by others
7. is angry a lot of the time
8. gets even when angered

Conduct Disorder

1. has stolen >1 time
2. a. lies to get out of doing things
    b. "cons" people
3. has broken into a car or building to steal
4. has skipped school >3 times
5. breaks curfew >1 time per month
6. has run away/stayed out all night >1 time or did not return for a long time
7. a. is a bully
    b. threatens other people
8. a. is avoided because he/she starts fights
    b. gets in trouble for fighting
9. has used a weapon in a fight >1 time
10. a. has hurt someone badly in a fight
    b. has hurt someone for no reason
11. has taken things from people by force
12. has damaged property
13. has set something on fire (>1 time or caused extensive damage)
14. has hurt or killed an animal for fun
15. a. has forcefully performed sexual activity on another
    b. has forced someone to perform sexual activity on him-/herself

Substance Abuse

1. a. has smoked cigarettes ≥2 times _____
    b. has smoked pot ≥2 times _____
    c. has smoked other drugs ≥2 times _____
2. has used alcohol _____
3. has used other drugs _____
4. has sniffed a substance ≥2 times _____

Specific Phobia

1. phobic object/situation: _____
2. when confronted with object/situation,
   a. gets uptight and scared, can't move
   b. cries, clings to parents, throws tantrums
3. a. avoids object/situation
   b. becomes nauseated, feels faint
4. a. fear interferes with (sleep, school, activities)
   b. feels *super* uncomfortable because of fear
5. a. is more scared of object/situation than peers
   b. fear seems silly to child

Social Phobia

1. a. is afraid of being around other people
   b. has fear of performing
2. feels super-uncomfortable when a/b occurs
3. a. tries to avoid social situations
   b. if unavoidable, feels awful
4. a. fear interferes with (sleep, school, activities)
   b. feels *super* uncomfortable because of fear
5. behavior seems silly to child

Separation Anxiety

1. a. cries, begs parent to stay home
   b. tries to stay home with parent at all times
2. a. worries about parent getting harmed
   b. fears parental harm if separated
3. fears personal harm when separated from parent
4. a. has difficulty going to school
   b. refuses to go to school
5. a. is afraid to be in room of house alone
   b. follows parent around the house
6. a. can't sleep if not with parent
   b. can't sleep away from home
7. a. has nightmares about separation
   b. has nightmares about parental loss
8. a. has stomach- or headaches before going to school
   b. gets ill when parent leaves him/her

Generalized Anxiety Disorder

1. worries more than other kids _____
2. a. has difficulty calming down
   b. can't let go of worry
3. when worried, feels edgy, tired, distractible, cranky; has tight muscles, poor sleep

Obsessive-Compulsive Disorder

A: Compulsions

1. does things over and over
2. a. feels behavior will improve things
   b. thinks that if he/she can't perform behavior, something bad will happen
3. feels that behavior does not make sense

B: Obsessions

1. a. has bothersome thoughts/ideas
   b. "sees" pictures in head repeatedly
   c. has to do something but never does it
2. a. tries to make bothersome thoughts go away
   b. tries to pretend that thoughts aren't there
   c. does other things to try to make thoughts go away

3. thoughts seem like child's own (as opposed to someone else putting thoughts in his/her mind)

C: Interference

1. a. thoughts/behaviors cause child discomfort
   b. thoughts/behaviors cause problems at (home, school, play)
   c. thoughts/behaviors interfere with daily routines (time spent daily: _____)

Stress Disorders—PTSD, ASD

A: Exposure

1. a. child experienced traumatic event _____
   b. child witnessed traumatic event happening to someone else _____
2. after event, felt helpless, shocked, horrified, like he/she was falling apart; was hard to calm down
3. how long ago did event happen? _____

B: Dissociation

1. after event, felt cut off from family/friends; felt fewer emotions, felt numb
2. felt out of touch, in a daze
3. felt that the world was not real
4. felt that self was no longer real
5. had trouble remembering event

C: Reexperiencing

1. a. replays event over and over in mind
   b. "sees" event happening again
   c. plays games about event over and over
2. a. has nightmares about event
   b. has nightmares but can't remember what they're about
3. a. "feels" event happening again
   b. acts like event is happening again
4. a. becomes upset when reminded of event
   b. becomes upset when in same physical setting in which event occurred
5. when reminded of event, gets anxious, achy, sweaty palms, breathing problems

D: Avoidance

1. a. avoids thinking/talking about event
   b. tries to be unafraid of anything
2. a. avoids activities that remind him/her of event
   b. avoids places that remind him/her of event
   c. avoids people that remind him/her of event
3. can't remember things about event
4. a. has decreased interest in things he/she used to enjoy
   b. has stopped doing things he/she used to enjoy
5. feels cut off from family/friends
6. feels fewer emotions; feels numb
7. a. feels he/she won't grow up
   b. feels he/she will die soon

E: Hyperarousal

1. a. has trouble falling asleep
   b. has trouble staying asleep
2. a. is harder to get along with
   b. is easily angered
3. has difficulty concentrating
4. is super-alert
5. is easily startled, jumpy

Anorexia

1. a. has lost weight by dieting
   b. tries to stay underweight
2. a. current weight and height _____
   b. weight and height when thinnest _____
3. a. is terrified of getting fat
   b. is afraid of gaining weight
   c. fears he/she won't stop eating if he/she starts
4. a. feels fat
   b. feels good/bad depending on weight
   c. thinks his/her weight is a problem
5. if she's started menstruation yet, amenorrhea?

Bulimia

1. eats lots of food in short time
2. feels he/she can't stop eating, only stops because
   _____
3. after eating, tries to lose weight by . . .
   a. not eating
   b. vomiting
   c. taking laxatives
   d. overexercising
4. a. is more weight-conscious than peers
   b. self-image depends on weight

Depression/Dysthymia

A: Dysphoric Mood

1. a. feels sad or depressed
   b. almost every day
   c. lasts most of the day
2. a. feels more irritable
   b. (i) fights (ii) cries (iii) temper
   c. almost every day
   d. lasts most of the day

B: Loss of Interest

1. a. used to have fun doing _____
   b. isn't fun anymore
2. a. wants to have fun but can't
   b. feels that nothing is fun anymore
   c. has lost interest in daily activities

C: Appetite Changes

1. a. has decreased appetite
   b. has lost weight without dieting
   c. clothes are too big now
2. a. has increased appetite
   b. has gained weight

D: Sleep Changes

1. goes to bed @ _____; wakes @ _____
   a. early insomnia
   b. middle insomnia
   c. late insomnia
2. a. naps a lot
   b. hypersomnia

E: Psychomotor Changes

1. a. can't sit still
   b. is fidgety
   c. wrings hands
   d. picks at him-/herself
2. a. takes longer to do things
   b. has difficulty doing anything

F: Low Energy

1. a. has no energy
   b. has to push self
   c. tires easily
   d. sits around, does nothing

G: Guilt

1. a. has bad thoughts about self
   b. feels down on self
   c. feels he/she is no good
   d. hates self
2. a. feels guilty a lot
   b. thinks he/she should be punished

H: Impaired Concentration

1. a. mind has slowed down
   b. forgets things more
   c. has trouble paying attention
   d. listens to teacher less than before
   e. grades have dropped
2. has difficulty making up mind

I: Hopelessness

1. a. feels that nothing good will happen in the future
   b. feels that things won't get any better
   c. feels that there's no hope for the future

J: Morbid/Suicidal Thoughts

1. a. thinks about death
   b. thinks about dead people/pets
2. a. wishes he/she were dead
   b. feels life isn't worth living
   c. has thought of suicide
   d. has thought of suicide plans
   e. has made suicide attempt

Mania/Hypomania

A: Elevated Mood

1. a. feels very, very good
   b. feels wonderful for no reason
   c. is "too high"
2. has discrete periods of irritability

B: Other Symptoms

1. a. believes he/she has special abilities
   b. believes he/she can do things better than anyone
2. a. has lots of energy, no need for sleep
   b. sleeps a lot less without feeling tired
   c. needs ≤3 hours of sleep to feel OK
3. a. has rapid, unstoppable speech
   b. talks so fast that family/friends worry
   c. is told he/she talks too much, too loudly
   d. talks too fast to be understood
4. a. thoughts race through mind
   b. thoughts come too fast to verbalize them all
   c. feels that mind is sped up, working too fast
5. has trouble focusing
6. a. does more things than usual
   b. has more energy than usual
   c. tries many different things
   d. family/friends are concerned
   e. is more active than usual
7. a. gets in trouble more
   b. does things he/she usually wouldn't
   c. gets hurt due to carelessness
   d. is a lot more interested in sex than usual

C: Interference

1. mood/behavior causes problems at (home, school, play)
2. mood/behavior is reason child is here

Enuresis

1. has wet bed after kindergarten
2. a. wets bed at night
   b. wets self during day
3. a. occurs when not sick
   b. is not due to effects of some medication

Encopresis

1. has had bowel movement outside of toilet after kindergarten
2. happens when not sick

Schizophrenia/Psychosis

A: Psychotic Symptoms

1. a. feels someone is out to harm him/her
   b. feels someone is trying to make him/her sick
   c. people seem to be against him/her
   d. people seem to talk about him/her
   e. people spy on him/her
2. a. eyes play tricks on him/her
   b. during daylight
   c. only when falling asleep
   d. ears play tricks on him/her
   e. voices talk about child's feelings/thoughts/acts
   f. voices talk to each other

> *Interviewer observed:*
> 3. *incoherent speech*
> 4. *disorganized or catatonic behavior*
> 5. *inappropriate affect or inability to speak*

B: Interference

1. since problems started, has more difficulty getting along with other people
2. since problems started, does worse in school
3. since problems started, is careless about looks/hygiene

Psychosocial Stressors

A: Child Abuse/Neglect

1. a. M/F criticizes child a lot
   b. M/F wishes child had never been born
   c. M/F says he/she hates child
2. a. M/F ignores child
   b. M/F misses child's doctor appointments
   c. M/F does not feed child
   d. M/F does not clothe child
3. a. child is spanked or hit
   b. child is sometimes spanked or hit for no reason
   c. child fears physical harm from M/F
   d. child has been bruised, sore, taken to doctor
4. child has been sexually abused
5. child has been made to go a whole day without food

B: Other Stressors

1. a. fighting within family
   b. among children
   c. between parents
   d. between parents and children
   e. fighting bothers child
2. child remembers parents' separation/divorce
3. a. family has money problems
   b. child is worried about money problems
4. a. family member is ill
   b. family member has been hospitalized
   c. child worries
5. a. family member drinks or uses drugs a lot
   b. child worries
6. a. family member has been in trouble with police
   b. child worries
7. a. someone close to child has gotten sick and died
   b. child was very upset
8. a. someone close to child was murdered
   b. child was very upset
   c. someone close to child was killed in an accident
   d. child was very upset
9. anything else we need to know so we can help you?
   _____
   _____
10. problems child thinks he/she needs help with?
    _____
    _____
11. anything in the interview that bothered you?
    _____
    _____

P-ChIPS Report Form

Child's Name: _____ Date: ____ / _____ / _____

Informant's Name: _____ Interviewer: _____

Informant's Relationship (circle one): Mother, Father, Stepmother, Stepfather, Guardian, Other _____

Attention-Deficit/Hyperactivity Disorder

A: Inattention

1. a. pays no attention to details
   b. makes careless mistakes on schoolwork
2. can't keep mind on what he/she is doing
3. a. has trouble listening to parent
   b. has trouble listening to teacher
4. has trouble finishing things
5. has trouble organizing self
6. avoids schoolwork
7. loses school supplies
8. a. is easily distracted
   b. teacher reports inattention/daydreaming
9. a. is forgetful
   b. teacher reports forgetfulness

B: Hyperactivity–Impulsivity

1. a. is often told to sit still
   b. is constantly moving hands/feet
2. a. has trouble staying in seat
   b. gets in trouble for getting out of chair
3. gets in trouble for running/climbing
4. a. is too loud when playing
   b. has difficulty playing quietly
5. teacher reports is always "on the go"
6. a. talks out of turn at school
   b. talks too much at home
7. blurts out answers to questions
8. a. pushes ahead in line
   b. can't wait for his/her turn in games
9. a. barges in on other kids' games
   b. pushes into others' groups
   c. interrupts busy people

Oppositional Defiant Disorder

1. a. loses temper when things don't go his/her way
   b. has frequent temper tantrums
2. a. talks back/argues with parents
   b. talks back/argues with teachers
3. a. breaks rules at home
   b. breaks rules at school
   c. refuses to follow teachers' directions
   d. disobeys direct orders
4. purposely "bugs" other people
5. blames others for his/her own mistakes
6. is easily angered by others
7. is angry a lot of the time
8. gets even when angered

Conduct Disorder

1. has stolen >1 time
2. a. lies to get out of doing things
   b. "cons" people
3. has broken into a car or building to steal
4. has skipped school >3 times
5. breaks curfew >1 time per month
6. has run away/stayed out all night >1 time *or* did not return for a long time
7. a. is a bully
   b. threatens other people
8. a. is avoided because he/she starts fights
   b. gets in trouble for fighting
9. has used a weapon in a fight >1 time
10. a. has hurt someone badly in a fight
    b. has hurt someone for no reason
11. has taken things from people by force
12. has damaged property
13. has set something on fire (>1 time *or* caused extensive damage)
14. has hurt or killed an animal for fun
15. a. has forcefully performed sexual activity on another
    b. has forced someone to perform sexual activity on him-/herself

Substance Abuse

1. a. has smoked cigarettes ≥2 times _____
   b. has smoked pot ≥2 times _____
   c. has smoked other drugs ≥2 times _____
2. has used alcohol _____
3. has used other drugs _____
4. has sniffed a substance ≥2 times _____

Specific Phobia

1. phobic object/situation: _____
2. when confronted with object/situation,
   a. gets uptight and scared, can't move
   b. cries, clings to parents, throws tantrums
3. a. avoids object/situation
   b. becomes nauseated, feels faint
4. a. fear interferes with (sleep, school, activities)
   b. feels *super* uncomfortable because of fear
5. a. is more scared of object/situation than peers
   b. fear seems silly to child

Social Phobia

1. a. is afraid of being around other people
   b. has fear of performing
2. feels super-uncomfortable when a/b occurs
3. a. tries to avoid social situations
   b. if unavoidable, feels awful
4. a. fear interferes with (sleep, school, activities)
   b. feels *super* uncomfortable because of fear
5. behavior seems silly to child

Separation Anxiety

1. a. cries, begs parent to stay home
   b. tries to stay home with parent at all times
2. a. worries about parent getting harmed
   b. fears parental harm if separated
3. fears personal harm when separated from parent
4. a. has difficulty going to school
   b. refuses to go to school
5. a. is afraid to be in room of house alone
   b. follows parent around the house
6. a. can't sleep if not with parent
   b. can't sleep away from home
7. a. has nightmares about separation
   b. has nightmares about parental loss
8. a. has stomach- or headaches before going to school
   b. gets ill when parent leaves him/her

Generalized Anxiety Disorder

1. worries more than other kids _____
2. a. has difficulty calming down
   b. can't let go of worry
3. when worried, feels edgy, tired, distractible, cranky; has tight muscles, poor sleep

Obsessive-Compulsive Disorder

A: Compulsions

1. does things over and over
2. a. feels behavior will improve things
   b. thinks that if he/she can't perform behavior, something bad will happen
3. feels that behavior does not make sense

B: Obsessions

1. a. has bothersome thoughts/ideas
   b. "sees" pictures in head repeatedly
   c. has to do something but never does it
2. a. tries to make bothersome thoughts go away
   b. tries to pretend that thoughts aren't there
   c. does other things to try to make thoughts go away

3. thoughts seem like child's own (as opposed to someone else putting thoughts in his/her mind)

C: Interference

1. a. thoughts/behaviors cause child discomfort
   b. thoughts/behaviors cause problems at (home, school, play)
   c. thoughts/behaviors interfere with daily routines (time spent daily: _____)

Stress Disorders—PTSD, ASD

A: Exposure

1. a. child experienced traumatic event _____
   b. child witnessed traumatic event happening to someone else _____
2. after event, felt helpless, shocked, horrified, like he/she was falling apart; was hard to calm down
3. how long ago did event happen? _____

B: Dissociation

1. after event, felt cut off from family/friends; felt fewer emotions, felt numb
2. felt out of touch, in a daze
3. felt that the world was not real
4. felt that self was no longer real
5. had trouble remembering event

C: Reexperiencing

1. a. replays event over and over in mind
   b. "sees" event happening again
   c. plays games about event over and over
2. a. has nightmares about event
   b. has nightmares but can't remember what they're about
3. a. "feels" event happening again
   b. acts like event is happening again
4. a. becomes upset when reminded of event
   b. becomes upset when in same physical setting in which event occurred
5. when reminded of event, gets anxious, achy, sweaty palms, breathing problems

D: Avoidance

1. a. avoids thinking/talking about event
   b. tries to be unafraid of anything
2. a. avoids activities that remind him/her of event
   b. avoids places that remind him/her of event
   c. avoids people that remind him/her of event
3. can't remember things about event
4. a. has decreased interest in things he/she used to enjoy
   b. has stopped doing things he/she used to enjoy
5. feels cut off from family/friends
6. feels fewer emotions; feels numb
7. a. feels he/she won't grow up
   b. feels he/she will die soon

E: Hyperarousal

1. a. has trouble falling asleep
   b. has trouble staying asleep
2. a. is harder to get along with
   b. is easily angered
3. has difficulty concentrating
4. is super-alert
5. is easily startled, jumpy

Anorexia

1. a. has lost weight by dieting
   b. tries to stay underweight
2. a. current weight and height _____
   b. weight and height when thinnest _____
3. a. is terrified of getting fat
   b. is afraid of gaining weight
   c. fears he/she won't stop eating if he/she starts
4. a. feels fat
   b. feels good/bad depending on weight
   c. thinks his/her weight is a problem
5. if she's started menstruation yet, amenorrhea?

Bulimia

1. eats lots of food in short time
2. feels he/she can't stop eating, only stops because
   _____
3. after eating, tries to lose weight by . . .
   a. not eating
   b. vomiting
   c. taking laxatives
   d. overexercising
4. a. is more weight-conscious than peers
   b. self-image depends on weight

Depression/Dysthymia

A: Dysphoric Mood

1. a. feels sad or depressed
   b. almost every day
   c. lasts most of the day
2. a. feels more irritable
   b. (i) fights (ii) cries (iii) temper
   c. almost every day
   d. lasts most of the day

B: Loss of Interest

1. a. used to have fun doing _____
   b. isn't fun anymore
2. a. wants to have fun but can't
   b. feels that nothing is fun anymore
   c. has lost interest in daily activities

C: Appetite Changes

1. a. has decreased appetite
   b. has lost weight without dieting
   c. clothes are too big now
2. a. has increased appetite
   b. has gained weight

D: Sleep Changes

1. goes to bed @ _____; wakes @ _____
   a. early insomnia
   b. middle insomnia
   c. late insomnia
2. a. naps a lot
   b. hypersomnia

E: Psychomotor Changes

1. a. can't sit still
   b. is fidgety
   c. wrings hands
   d. picks at him-/herself
2. a. takes longer to do things
   b. has difficulty doing anything

F: Low Energy

1. a. has no energy
   b. has to push self

c. tires easily
d. sits around, does nothing

G: Guilt

1. a. has bad thoughts about self
   b. feels down on self
   c. feels he/she is no good
   d. hates self
2. a. feels guilty a lot
   b. thinks he/she should be punished

H: Impaired Concentration

1. a. mind has slowed down
   b. forgets things more
   c. has trouble paying attention
   d. listens to teacher less than before
   e. grades have dropped
2. has difficulty making up mind

I: Hopelessness

1. a. feels that nothing good will happen in the future
   b. feels that things won't get any better
   c. feels that there's no hope for the future

J: Morbid/Suicidal Thoughts

1. a. thinks about death
   b. thinks about dead people/pets
2. a. wishes he/she were dead
   b. feels life isn't worth living
   c. has thought of suicide
   d. has thought of suicide plans
   e. has made suicide attempt

Mania/Hypomania

A: Elevated Mood

1. a. feels very, very good
   b. feels wonderful for no reason
   c. is "too high"
2. has discrete periods of irritability

B: Other Symptoms

1. a. believes he/she has special abilities
   b. believes he/she can do things better than anyone
2. a. has lots of energy, no need for sleep
   b. sleeps a lot less without feeling tired
   c. needs ≤3 hours of sleep to feel OK
3. a. has rapid, unstoppable speech
   b. talks so fast that family/friends worry
   c. is told he/she talks too much, too loudly
   d. talks too fast to be understood
4. a. thoughts race through mind
   b. thoughts come too fast to verbalize them all
   c. feels that mind is sped up, working too fast
5. has trouble focusing
6. a. does more things than usual
   b. has more energy than usual
   c. tries many different things
   d. family/friends are concerned
   e. is more active than usual
7. a. gets in trouble more
   b. does things he/she usually wouldn't
   c. gets hurt due to carelessness
   d. is a lot more interested in sex than usual

C: Interference

1. mood/behavior causes problems at (home, school, play)
2. mood/behavior is reason child is here

Enuresis

1. has wet bed after kindergarten
2. a. wets bed at night
   b. wets self during day
3. a. occurs when not sick
   b. is not due to effects of some medication

Encopresis

1. has had bowel movement outside of toilet after kindergarten
2. happens when not sick

Schizophrenia/Psychosis

A: Psychotic Symptoms

1. a. feels someone is out to harm him/her
   b. feels someone is trying to make him/her sick
   c. people seem to be against him/her
   d. people seem to talk about him/her
   e. people spy on him/her
2. a. eyes play tricks on him/her
   b. during daylight
   c. only when falling asleep
   d. ears play tricks on him/her
   e. voices talk about child's feelings/thoughts/acts
   f. voices talk to each other

Interviewer observed:
3. *incoherent speech*
4. *disorganized or catatonic behavior*
5. *inappropriate affect or inability to speak*

B: Interference

1. since problems started, has more difficulty getting along with other people
2. since problems started, does worse in school
3. since problems started, is careless about looks/hygiene

Psychosocial Stressors

A: Child Abuse/Neglect

1. a. M/F criticizes child a lot
   b. M/F wishes child had never been born
   c. M/F says he/she hates child
2. a. M/F ignores child
   b. M/F misses child's doctor appointments
   c. M/F does not feed child
   d. M/F does not clothe child
3. a. child is spanked or hit
   b. child is sometimes spanked or hit for no reason
   c. child fears physical harm from M/F
   d. child has been bruised, sore, taken to doctor
4. child has been sexually abused
5. child has been made to go a whole day without food

B: Other Stressors

1. a. fighting within family
   b. among children
   c. between parents
   d. between parents and children
   e. fighting bothers child
2. child remembers parents' separation/divorce
3. a. family has money problems
   b. child is worried about money problems
4. a. family member is ill
   b. family member has been hospitalized
   c. child worries
5. a. family member drinks or uses drugs a lot
   b. child worries
6. a. family member has been in trouble with police
   b. child worries
7. a. someone close to child has gotten sick and died
   b. child was very upset
8. a. someone close to child was murdered
   b. child was very upset
   c. someone close to child was killed in an accident
   d. child was very upset
9. anything else we need to know so we can help you?
   _____
   _____
10. problems child thinks he/she needs help with?
   _____
   _____
11. anything in the interview that bothered you?
   _____
   _____

P-ChIPS Report Form

Child's Name: _____ Date: _____ / _____ / _____

Informant's Name: _____ Interviewer: _____

Informant's Relationship (circle one): Mother, Father, Stepmother, Stepfather, Guardian, Other _____

Attention-Deficit/Hyperactivity Disorder

A: Inattention
1. a. pays no attention to details
   b. makes careless mistakes on schoolwork
2. can't keep mind on what he/she is doing
3. a. has trouble listening to parent
   b. has trouble listening to teacher
4. has trouble finishing things
5. has trouble organizing self
6. avoids schoolwork
7. loses school supplies
8. a. is easily distracted
   b. teacher reports inattention/daydreaming
9. a. is forgetful
   b. teacher reports forgetfulness

B: Hyperactivity–Impulsivity
1. a. is often told to sit still
   b. is constantly moving hands/feet
2. a. has trouble staying in seat
   b. gets in trouble for getting out of chair
3. gets in trouble for running/climbing
4. a. is too loud when playing
   b. has difficulty playing quietly
5. teacher reports is always "on the go"
6. a. talks out of turn at school
   b. talks too much at home
7. blurts out answers to questions
8. a. pushes ahead in line
   b. can't wait for his/her turn in games
9. a. barges in on other kids' games
   b. pushes into others' groups
   c. interrupts busy people

Oppositional Defiant Disorder
1. a. loses temper when things don't go his/her way
   b. has frequent temper tantrums
2. a. talks back/argues with parents
   b. talks back/argues with teachers
3. a. breaks rules at home
   b. breaks rules at school
   c. refuses to follow teachers' directions
   d. disobeys direct orders
4. purposely "bugs" other people
5. blames others for his/her own mistakes
6. is easily angered by others
7. is angry a lot of the time
8. gets even when angered

Conduct Disorder
1. has stolen >1 time
2. a. lies to get out of doing things
   b. "cons" people
3. has broken into a car or building to steal
4. has skipped school >3 times
5. breaks curfew >1 time per month
6. has run away/stayed out all night >1 time *or* did not return for a long time
7. a. is a bully
   b. threatens other people
8. a. is avoided because he/she starts fights
   b. gets in trouble for fighting
9. has used a weapon in a fight >1 time
10. a. has hurt someone badly in a fight
    b. has hurt someone for no reason
11. has taken things from people by force
12. has damaged property
13. has set something on fire (>1 time *or* caused extensive damage)
14. has hurt or killed an animal for fun
15. a. has forcefully performed sexual activity on another
    b. has forced someone to perform sexual activity on him-/herself

Substance Abuse
1. a. has smoked cigarettes ≥2 times _____
   b. has smoked pot ≥2 times _____
   c. has smoked other drugs ≥2 times _____
2. has used alcohol _____
3. has used other drugs _____
4. has sniffed a substance ≥2 times _____

Specific Phobia

1. phobic object/situation: _____
2. when confronted with object/situation,
   a. gets uptight and scared, can't move
   b. cries, clings to parents, throws tantrums
3. a. avoids object/situation
   b. becomes nauseated, feels faint
4. a. fear interferes with (sleep, school, activities)
   b. feels *super* uncomfortable because of fear
5. a. is more scared of object/situation than peers
   b. fear seems silly to child

Social Phobia

1. a. is afraid of being around other people
   b. has fear of performing
2. feels super-uncomfortable when a/b occurs
3. a. tries to avoid social situations
   b. if unavoidable, feels awful
4. a. fear interferes with (sleep, school, activities)
   b. feels *super* uncomfortable because of fear
5. behavior seems silly to child

Separation Anxiety

1. a. cries, begs parent to stay home
   b. tries to stay home with parent at all times
2. a. worries about parent getting harmed
   b. fears parental harm if separated
3. fears personal harm when separated from parent
4. a. has difficulty going to school
   b. refuses to go to school
5. a. is afraid to be in room of house alone
   b. follows parent around the house
6. a. can't sleep if not with parent
   b. can't sleep away from home
7. a. has nightmares about separation
   b. has nightmares about parental loss
8. a. has stomach- or headaches before going to school
   b. gets ill when parent leaves him/her

Generalized Anxiety Disorder

1. worries more than other kids _____
2. a. has difficulty calming down
   b. can't let go of worry
3. when worried, feels edgy, tired, distractible, cranky; has tight muscles, poor sleep

Obsessive-Compulsive Disorder

A: Compulsions

1. does things over and over
2. a. feels behavior will improve things
   b. thinks that if he/she can't perform behavior, something bad will happen
3. feels that behavior does not make sense

B: Obsessions

1. a. has bothersome thoughts/ideas
   b. "sees" pictures in head repeatedly
   c. has to do something but never does it
2. a. tries to make bothersome thoughts go away
   b. tries to pretend that thoughts aren't there
   c. does other things to try to make thoughts go away

3. thoughts seem like child's own (as opposed to someone else putting thoughts in his/her mind)

C: Interference

1. a. thoughts/behaviors cause child discomfort
   b. thoughts/behaviors cause problems at (home, school, play)
   c. thoughts/behaviors interfere with daily routines (time spent daily: _____)

Stress Disorders—PTSD, ASD

A: Exposure

1. a. child experienced traumatic event _____
   b. child witnessed traumatic event happening to someone else _____
2. after event, felt helpless, shocked, horrified, like he/she was falling apart; was hard to calm down
3. how long ago did event happen? _____

B: Dissociation

1. after event, felt cut off from family/friends; felt fewer emotions, felt numb
2. felt out of touch, in a daze
3. felt that the world was not real
4. felt that self was no longer real
5. had trouble remembering event

C: Reexperiencing

1. a. replays event over and over in mind
   b. "sees" event happening again
   c. plays games about event over and over
2. a. has nightmares about event
   b. has nightmares but can't remember what they're about
3. a. "feels" event happening again
   b. acts like event is happening again
4. a. becomes upset when reminded of event
   b. becomes upset when in same physical setting in which event occurred
5. when reminded of event, gets anxious, achy, sweaty palms, breathing problems

D: Avoidance

1. a. avoids thinking/talking about event
   b. tries to be unafraid of anything
2. a. avoids activities that remind him/her of event
   b. avoids places that remind him/her of event
   c. avoids people that remind him/her of event
3. can't remember things about event
4. a. has decreased interest in things he/she used to enjoy
   b. has stopped doing things he/she used to enjoy
5. feels cut off from family/friends
6. feels fewer emotions; feels numb
7. a. feels he/she won't grow up
   b. feels he/she will die soon

E: Hyperarousal

1. a. has trouble falling asleep
   b. has trouble staying asleep
2. a. is harder to get along with
   b. is easily angered
3. has difficulty concentrating
4. is super-alert
5. is easily startled, jumpy

Anorexia

1. a. has lost weight by dieting
   b. tries to stay underweight
2. a. current weight and height _____
   b. weight and height when thinnest _____
3. a. is terrified of getting fat
   b. is afraid of gaining weight
   c. fears he/she won't stop eating if he/she starts
4. a. feels fat
   b. feels good/bad depending on weight
   c. thinks his/her weight is a problem
5. if she's started menstruation yet, amenorrhea?

Bulimia

1. eats lots of food in short time
2. feels he/she can't stop eating, only stops because
   _____
3. after eating, tries to lose weight by . . .
   a. not eating
   b. vomiting
   c. taking laxatives
   d. overexercising
4. a. is more weight-conscious than peers
   b. self-image depends on weight

Depression/Dysthymia

A: Dysphoric Mood
1. a. feels sad or depressed
   b. almost every day
   c. lasts most of the day
2. a. feels more irritable
   b. (i) fights (ii) cries (iii) temper
   c. almost every day
   d. lasts most of the day

B: Loss of Interest
1. a. used to have fun doing _____
   b. isn't fun anymore
2. a. wants to have fun but can't
   b. feels that nothing is fun anymore
   c. has lost interest in daily activities

C: Appetite Changes
1. a. has decreased appetite
   b. has lost weight without dieting
   c. clothes are too big now
2. a. has increased appetite
   b. has gained weight

D: Sleep Changes
1. goes to bed @ _____; wakes @ _____
   a. early insomnia
   b. middle insomnia
   c. late insomnia
2. a. naps a lot
   b. hypersomnia

E: Psychomotor Changes
1. a. can't sit still
   b. is fidgety
   c. wrings hands
   d. picks at him-/herself
2. a. takes longer to do things
   b. has difficulty doing anything

F: Low Energy
1. a. has no energy
   b. has to push self
c. tires easily
d. sits around, does nothing

G: Guilt
1. a. has bad thoughts about self
   b. feels down on self
   c. feels he/she is no good
   d. hates self
2. a. feels guilty a lot
   b. thinks he/she should be punished

H: Impaired Concentration
1. a. mind has slowed down
   b. forgets things more
   c. has trouble paying attention
   d. listens to teacher less than before
   e. grades have dropped
2. has difficulty making up mind

I: Hopelessness
1. a. feels that nothing good will happen in the future
   b. feels that things won't get any better
   c. feels that there's no hope for the future

J: Morbid/Suicidal Thoughts
1. a. thinks about death
   b. thinks about dead people/pets
2. a. wishes he/she were dead
   b. feels life isn't worth living
   c. has thought of suicide
   d. has thought of suicide plans
   e. has made suicide attempt

Mania/Hypomania

A: Elevated Mood
1. a. feels very, very good
   b. feels wonderful for no reason
   c. is "too high"
2. has discrete periods of irritability

B: Other Symptoms
1. a. believes he/she has special abilities
   b. believes he/she can do things better than anyone
2. a. has lots of energy, no need for sleep
   b. sleeps a lot less without feeling tired
   c. needs ≤3 hours of sleep to feel OK
3. a. has rapid, unstoppable speech
   b. talks so fast that family/friends worry
   c. is told he/she talks too much, too loudly
   d. talks too fast to be understood
4. a. thoughts race through mind
   b. thoughts come too fast to verbalize them all
   c. feels that mind is sped up, working too fast
5. has trouble focusing
6. a. does more things than usual
   b. has more energy than usual
   c. tries many different things
   d. family/friends are concerned
   e. is more active than usual
7. a. gets in trouble more
   b. does things he/she usually wouldn't
   c. gets hurt due to carelessness
   d. is a lot more interested in sex than usual

C: Interference
1. mood/behavior causes problems at (home, school, play)
2. mood/behavior is reason child is here

Enuresis

1. has wet bed after kindergarten
2. a. wets bed at night
   b. wets self during day
3. a. occurs when not sick
   b. is not due to effects of some medication

Encopresis

1. has had bowel movement outside of toilet after kindergarten
2. happens when not sick

Schizophrenia/Psychosis

A: Psychotic Symptoms

1. a. feels someone is out to harm him/her
   b. feels someone is trying to make him/her sick
   c. people seem to be against him/her
   d. people seem to talk about him/her
   e. people spy on him/her
2. a. eyes play tricks on him/her
   b. during daylight
   c. only when falling asleep
   d. ears play tricks on him/her
   e. voices talk about child's feelings/thoughts/acts
   f. voices talk to each other

Interviewer observed:
3. *incoherent speech*
4. *disorganized or catatonic behavior*
5. *inappropriate affect or inability to speak*

B: Interference

1. since problems started, has more difficulty getting along with other people
2. since problems started, does worse in school
3. since problems started, is careless about looks/ hygiene

Psychosocial Stressors

A: Child Abuse/Neglect

1. a. M/F criticizes child a lot
   b. M/F wishes child had never been born
   c. M/F says he/she hates child
2. a. M/F ignores child
   b. M/F misses child's doctor appointments
   c. M/F does not feed child
   d. M/F does not clothe child
3. a. child is spanked or hit
   b. child is sometimes spanked or hit for no reason
   c. child fears physical harm from M/F
   d. child has been bruised, sore, taken to doctor
4. child has been sexually abused
5. child has been made to go a whole day without food

B: Other Stressors

1. a. fighting within family
   b. among children
   c. between parents
   d. between parents and children
   e. fighting bothers child
2. child remembers parents' separation/divorce
3. a. family has money problems
   b. child is worried about money problems
4. a. family member is ill
   b. family member has been hospitalized
   c. child worries
5. a. family member drinks or uses drugs a lot
   b. child worries
6. a. family member has been in trouble with police
   b. child worries
7. a. someone close to child has gotten sick and died
   b. child was very upset
8. a. someone close to child was murdered
   b. child was very upset
   c. someone close to child was killed in an accident
   d. child was very upset
9. anything else we need to know so we can help you?
   _____
   _____
10. problems child thinks he/she needs help with?
    _____
    _____
11. anything in the interview that bothered you?
    _____
    _____

P-ChIPS Report Form

Child's Name: _____ Date: _____ / _____ / _____

Informant's Name: _____ Interviewer: _____

Informant's Relationship (circle one): Mother, Father, Stepmother, Stepfather, Guardian, Other _____

Attention-Deficit/Hyperactivity Disorder

A: Inattention

1. a. pays no attention to details
    b. makes careless mistakes on schoolwork
2. can't keep mind on what he/she is doing
3. a. has trouble listening to parent
    b. has trouble listening to teacher
4. has trouble finishing things
5. has trouble organizing self
6. avoids schoolwork
7. loses school supplies
8. a. is easily distracted
    b. teacher reports inattention/daydreaming
9. a. is forgetful
    b. teacher reports forgetfulness

B: Hyperactivity–Impulsivity

1. a. is often told to sit still
    b. is constantly moving hands/feet
2. a. has trouble staying in seat
    b. gets in trouble for getting out of chair
3. gets in trouble for running/climbing
4. a. is too loud when playing
    b. has difficulty playing quietly
5. teacher reports is always "on the go"
6. a. talks out of turn at school
    b. talks too much at home
7. blurts out answers to questions
8. a. pushes ahead in line
    b. can't wait for his/her turn in games
9. a. barges in on other kids' games
    b. pushes into others' groups
    c. interrupts busy people

Oppositional Defiant Disorder

1. a. loses temper when things don't go his/her way
    b. has frequent temper tantrums
2. a. talks back/argues with parents
    b. talks back/argues with teachers
3. a. breaks rules at home
    b. breaks rules at school
    c. refuses to follow teachers' directions
    d. disobeys direct orders
4. purposely "bugs" other people
5. blames others for his/her own mistakes
6. is easily angered by others
7. is angry a lot of the time
8. gets even when angered

Conduct Disorder

1. has stolen >1 time
2. a. lies to get out of doing things
    b. "cons" people
3. has broken into a car or building to steal
4. has skipped school >3 times
5. breaks curfew >1 time per month
6. has run away/stayed out all night >1 time *or* did not return for a long time
7. a. is a bully
    b. threatens other people
8. a. is avoided because he/she starts fights
    b. gets in trouble for fighting
9. has used a weapon in a fight >1 time
10. a. has hurt someone badly in a fight
    b. has hurt someone for no reason
11. has taken things from people by force
12. has damaged property
13. has set something on fire (>1 time *or* caused extensive damage)
14. has hurt or killed an animal for fun
15. a. has forcefully performed sexual activity on another
    b. has forced someone to perform sexual activity on him-/herself

Substance Abuse

1. a. has smoked cigarettes ≥2 times _____
    b. has smoked pot ≥2 times _____
    c. has smoked other drugs ≥2 times _____
2. has used alcohol _____
3. has used other drugs _____
4. has sniffed a substance ≥2 times _____

Specific Phobia

1. phobic object/situation: _____
2. when confronted with object/situation,
   a. gets uptight and scared, can't move
   b. cries, clings to parents, throws tantrums
3. a. avoids object/situation
   b. becomes nauseated, feels faint
4. a. fear interferes with (sleep, school, activities)
   b. feels *super* uncomfortable because of fear
5. a. is more scared of object/situation than peers
   b. fear seems silly to child

Social Phobia

1. a. is afraid of being around other people
   b. has fear of performing
2. feels super-uncomfortable when a/b occurs
3. a. tries to avoid social situations
   b. if unavoidable, feels awful
4. a. fear interferes with (sleep, school, activities)
   b. feels *super* uncomfortable because of fear
5. behavior seems silly to child

Separation Anxiety

1. a. cries, begs parent to stay home
   b. tries to stay home with parent at all times
2. a. worries about parent getting harmed
   b. fears parental harm if separated
3. fears personal harm when separated from parent
4. a. has difficulty going to school
   b. refuses to go to school
5. a. is afraid to be in room of house alone
   b. follows parent around the house
6. a. can't sleep if not with parent
   b. can't sleep away from home
7. a. has nightmares about separation
   b. has nightmares about parental loss
8. a. has stomach- or headaches before going to school
   b. gets ill when parent leaves him/her

Generalized Anxiety Disorder

1. worries more than other kids _____
2. a. has difficulty calming down
   b. can't let go of worry
3. when worried, feels edgy, tired, distractible, cranky; has tight muscles, poor sleep

Obsessive-Compulsive Disorder

A: Compulsions

1. does things over and over
2. a. feels behavior will improve things
   b. thinks that if he/she can't perform behavior, something bad will happen
3. feels that behavior does not make sense

B: Obsessions

1. a. has bothersome thoughts/ideas
   b. "sees" pictures in head repeatedly
   c. has to do something but never does it
2. a. tries to make bothersome thoughts go away
   b. tries to pretend that thoughts aren't there
   c. does other things to try to make thoughts go away
3. thoughts seem like child's own (as opposed to someone else putting thoughts in his/her mind)

C: Interference

1. a. thoughts/behaviors cause child discomfort
   b. thoughts/behaviors cause problems at (home, school, play)
   c. thoughts/behaviors interfere with daily routines (time spent daily: _____)

Stress Disorders—PTSD, ASD

A: Exposure

1. a. child experienced traumatic event _____
   b. child witnessed traumatic event happening to someone else _____
2. after event, felt helpless, shocked, horrified, like he/she was falling apart; was hard to calm down
3. how long ago did event happen? _____

B: Dissociation

1. after event, felt cut off from family/friends; felt fewer emotions, felt numb
2. felt out of touch, in a daze
3. felt that the world was not real
4. felt that self was no longer real
5. had trouble remembering event

C: Reexperiencing

1. a. replays event over and over in mind
   b. "sees" event happening again
   c. plays games about event over and over
2. a. has nightmares about event
   b. has nightmares but can't remember what they're about
3. a. "feels" event happening again
   b. acts like event is happening again
4. a. becomes upset when reminded of event
   b. becomes upset when in same physical setting in which event occurred
5. when reminded of event, gets anxious, achy, sweaty palms, breathing problems

D: Avoidance

1. a. avoids thinking/talking about event
   b. tries to be unafraid of anything
2. a. avoids activities that remind him/her of event
   b. avoids places that remind him/her of event
   c. avoids people that remind him/her of event
3. can't remember things about event
4. a. has decreased interest in things he/she used to enjoy
   b. has stopped doing things he/she used to enjoy
5. feels cut off from family/friends
6. feels fewer emotions; feels numb
7. a. feels he/she won't grow up
   b. feels he/she will die soon

E: Hyperarousal

1. a. has trouble falling asleep
   b. has trouble staying asleep
2. a. is harder to get along with
   b. is easily angered
3. has difficulty concentrating
4. is super-alert
5. is easily startled, jumpy

Anorexia

1. a. has lost weight by dieting
   b. tries to stay underweight
2. a. current weight and height _____
   b. weight and height when thinnest _____
3. a. is terrified of getting fat
   b. is afraid of gaining weight
   c. fears he/she won't stop eating if he/she starts
4. a. feels fat
   b. feels good/bad depending on weight
   c. thinks his/her weight is a problem
5. if she's started menstruation yet, amenorrhea?

Bulimia

1. eats lots of food in short time
2. feels he/she can't stop eating, only stops because

   _____
3. after eating, tries to lose weight by . . .
   a. not eating
   b. vomiting
   c. taking laxatives
   d. overexercising
4. a. is more weight-conscious than peers
   b. self-image depends on weight

Depression/Dysthymia

A: Dysphoric Mood

1. a. feels sad or depressed
   b. almost every day
   c. lasts most of the day
2. a. feels more irritable
   b. (i) fights (ii) cries (iii) temper
   c. almost every day
   d. lasts most of the day

B: Loss of Interest

1. a. used to have fun doing _____
   b. isn't fun anymore
2. a. wants to have fun but can't
   b. feels that nothing is fun anymore
   c. has lost interest in daily activities

C: Appetite Changes

1. a. has decreased appetite
   b. has lost weight without dieting
   c. clothes are too big now
2. a. has increased appetite
   b. has gained weight

D: Sleep Changes

1. goes to bed @ _____; wakes @ _____
   a. early insomnia
   b. middle insomnia
   c. late insomnia
2. a. naps a lot
   b. hypersomnia

E: Psychomotor Changes

1. a. can't sit still
   b. is fidgety
   c. wrings hands
   d. picks at him-/herself
2. a. takes longer to do things
   b. has difficulty doing anything

F: Low Energy

1. a. has no energy
   b. has to push self
   c. tires easily
   d. sits around, does nothing

G: Guilt

1. a. has bad thoughts about self
   b. feels down on self
   c. feels he/she is no good
   d. hates self
2. a. feels guilty a lot
   b. thinks he/she should be punished

H: Impaired Concentration

1. a. mind has slowed down
   b. forgets things more
   c. has trouble paying attention
   d. listens to teacher less than before
   e. grades have dropped
2. has difficulty making up mind

I: Hopelessness

1. a. feels that nothing good will happen in the future
   b. feels that things won't get any better
   c. feels that there's no hope for the future

J: Morbid/Suicidal Thoughts

1. a. thinks about death
   b. thinks about dead people/pets
2. a. wishes he/she were dead
   b. feels life isn't worth living
   c. has thought of suicide
   d. has thought of suicide plans
   e. has made suicide attempt

Mania/Hypomania

A: Elevated Mood

1. a. feels very, very good
   b. feels wonderful for no reason
   c. is "too high"
2. has discrete periods of irritability

B: Other Symptoms

1. a. believes he/she has special abilities
   b. believes he/she can do things better than anyone
2. a. has lots of energy, no need for sleep
   b. sleeps a lot less without feeling tired
   c. needs ≤3 hours of sleep to feel OK
3. a. has rapid, unstoppable speech
   b. talks so fast that family/friends worry
   c. is told he/she talks too much, too loudly
   d. talks too fast to be understood
4. a. thoughts race through mind
   b. thoughts come too fast to verbalize them all
   c. feels that mind is sped up, working too fast
5. has trouble focusing
6. a. does more things than usual
   b. has more energy than usual
   c. tries many different things
   d. family/friends are concerned
   e. is more active than usual
7. a. gets in trouble more
   b. does things he/she usually wouldn't
   c. gets hurt due to carelessness
   d. is a lot more interested in sex than usual

C: Interference

1. mood/behavior causes problems at (home, school, play)
2. mood/behavior is reason child is here

Enuresis

1. has wet bed after kindergarten
2. a. wets bed at night
   b. wets self during day
3. a. occurs when not sick
   b. is not due to effects of some medication

Encopresis

1. has had bowel movement outside of toilet after kindergarten
2. happens when not sick

Schizophrenia/Psychosis

A: Psychotic Symptoms

1. a. feels someone is out to harm him/her
   b. feels someone is trying to make him/her sick
   c. people seem to be against him/her
   d. people seem to talk about him/her
   e. people spy on him/her
2. a. eyes play tricks on him/her
   b. during daylight
   c. only when falling asleep
   d. ears play tricks on him/her
   e. voices talk about child's feelings/thoughts/acts
   f. voices talk to each other

> **Interviewer observed:**
> 3. incoherent speech
> 4. disorganized or catatonic behavior
> 5. inappropriate affect or inability to speak

B: Interference

1. since problems started, has more difficulty getting along with other people
2. since problems started, does worse in school
3. since problems started, is careless about looks/ hygiene

Psychosocial Stressors

A: Child Abuse/Neglect

1. a. M/F criticizes child a lot
   b. M/F wishes child had never been born
   c. M/F says he/she hates child
2. a. M/F ignores child
   b. M/F misses child's doctor appointments
   c. M/F does not feed child
   d. M/F does not clothe child
3. a. child is spanked or hit
   b. child is sometimes spanked or hit for no reason
   c. child fears physical harm from M/F
   d. child has been bruised, sore, taken to doctor
4. child has been sexually abused
5. child has been made to go a whole day without food

B: Other Stressors

1. a. fighting within family
   b. among children
   c. between parents
   d. between parents and children
   e. fighting bothers child
2. child remembers parents' separation/divorce
3. a. family has money problems
   b. child is worried about money problems
4. a. family member is ill
   b. family member has been hospitalized
   c. child worries
5. a. family member drinks or uses drugs a lot
   b. child worries
6. a. family member has been in trouble with police
   b. child worries
7. a. someone close to child has gotten sick and died
   b. child was very upset
8. a. someone close to child was murdered
   b. child was very upset
   c. someone close to child was killed in an accident
   d. child was very upset
9. anything else we need to know so we can help you?
   _____
   _____
10. problems child thinks he/she needs help with?
    _____
    _____
11. anything in the interview that bothered you?
    _____
    _____

P-ChIPS Report Form

Child's Name: _____ Date: ____ / _____ / _____

Informant's Name: _____ Interviewer: _____

Informant's Relationship (circle one): Mother, Father, Stepmother, Stepfather, Guardian, Other _____

Attention-Deficit/Hyperactivity Disorder

A: Inattention

1. a. pays no attention to details
   b. makes careless mistakes on schoolwork
2. can't keep mind on what he/she is doing
3. a. has trouble listening to parent
   b. has trouble listening to teacher
4. has trouble finishing things
5. has trouble organizing self
6. avoids schoolwork
7. loses school supplies
8. a. is easily distracted
   b. teacher reports inattention/daydreaming
9. a. is forgetful
   b. teacher reports forgetfulness

B: Hyperactivity–Impulsivity

1. a. is often told to sit still
   b. is constantly moving hands/feet
2. a. has trouble staying in seat
   b. gets in trouble for getting out of chair
3. gets in trouble for running/climbing
4. a. is too loud when playing
   b. has difficulty playing quietly
5. teacher reports is always "on the go"
6. a. talks out of turn at school
   b. talks too much at home
7. blurts out answers to questions
8. a. pushes ahead in line
   b. can't wait for his/her turn in games
9. a. barges in on other kids' games
   b. pushes into others' groups
   c. interrupts busy people

Oppositional Defiant Disorder

1. a. loses temper when things don't go his/her way
   b. has frequent temper tantrums
2. a. talks back/argues with parents
   b. talks back/argues with teachers
3. a. breaks rules at home
   b. breaks rules at school
   c. refuses to follow teachers' directions
   d. disobeys direct orders
4. purposely "bugs" other people
5. blames others for his/her own mistakes
6. is easily angered by others
7. is angry a lot of the time
8. gets even when angered

Conduct Disorder

1. has stolen >1 time
2. a. lies to get out of doing things
   b. "cons" people
3. has broken into a car or building to steal
4. has skipped school >3 times
5. breaks curfew >1 time per month
6. has run away/stayed out all night >1 time *or* did not return for a long time
7. a. is a bully
   b. threatens other people
8. a. is avoided because he/she starts fights
   b. gets in trouble for fighting
9. has used a weapon in a fight >1 time
10. a. has hurt someone badly in a fight
    b. has hurt someone for no reason
11. has taken things from people by force
12. has damaged property
13. has set something on fire (>1 time *or* caused extensive damage)
14. has hurt or killed an animal for fun
15. a. has forcefully performed sexual activity on another
    b. has forced someone to perform sexual activity on him-/herself

Substance Abuse

1. a. has smoked cigarettes ≥2 times _____
   b. has smoked pot ≥2 times _____
   c. has smoked other drugs ≥2 times _____
2. has used alcohol _____
3. has used other drugs _____
4. has sniffed a substance ≥2 times _____

Specific Phobia

1. phobic object/situation: _____
2. when confronted with object/situation,
   a. gets uptight and scared, can't move
   b. cries, clings to parents, throws tantrums
3. a. avoids object/situation
   b. becomes nauseated, feels faint
4. a. fear interferes with (sleep, school, activities)
   b. feels *super* uncomfortable because of fear
5. a. is more scared of object/situation than peers
   b. fear seems silly to child

Social Phobia

1. a. is afraid of being around other people
   b. has fear of performing
2. feels super-uncomfortable when a/b occurs
3. a. tries to avoid social situations
   b. if unavoidable, feels awful
4. a. fear interferes with (sleep, school, activities)
   b. feels *super* uncomfortable because of fear
5. behavior seems silly to child

Separation Anxiety

1. a. cries, begs parent to stay home
   b. tries to stay home with parent at all times
2. a. worries about parent getting harmed
   b. fears parental harm if separated
3. fears personal harm when separated from parent
4. a. has difficulty going to school
   b. refuses to go to school
5. a. is afraid to be in room of house alone
   b. follows parent around the house
6. a. can't sleep if not with parent
   b. can't sleep away from home
7. a. has nightmares about separation
   b. has nightmares about parental loss
8. a. has stomach- or headaches before going to school
   b. gets ill when parent leaves him/her

Generalized Anxiety Disorder

1. worries more than other kids _____
2. a. has difficulty calming down
   b. can't let go of worry
3. when worried, feels edgy, tired, distractible, cranky; has tight muscles, poor sleep

Obsessive-Compulsive Disorder

A: Compulsions

1. does things over and over
2. a. feels behavior will improve things
   b. thinks that if he/she can't perform behavior, something bad will happen
3. feels that behavior does not make sense

B: Obsessions

1. a. has bothersome thoughts/ideas
   b. "sees" pictures in head repeatedly
   c. has to do something but never does it
2. a. tries to make bothersome thoughts go away
   b. tries to pretend that thoughts aren't there
   c. does other things to try to make thoughts go away

3. thoughts seem like child's own (as opposed to someone else putting thoughts in his/her mind)

C: Interference

1. a. thoughts/behaviors cause child discomfort
   b. thoughts/behaviors cause problems at (home, school, play)
   c. thoughts/behaviors interfere with daily routines (time spent daily: _____)

Stress Disorders—PTSD, ASD

A: Exposure

1. a. child experienced traumatic event _____
   b. child witnessed traumatic event happening to someone else _____
2. after event, felt helpless, shocked, horrified, like he/she was falling apart; was hard to calm down
3. how long ago did event happen? _____

B: Dissociation

1. after event, felt cut off from family/friends; felt fewer emotions, felt numb
2. felt out of touch, in a daze
3. felt that the world was not real
4. felt that self was no longer real
5. had trouble remembering event

C: Reexperiencing

1. a. replays event over and over in mind
   b. "sees" event happening again
   c. plays games about event over and over
2. a. has nightmares about event
   b. has nightmares but can't remember what they're about
3. a. "feels" event happening again
   b. acts like event is happening again
4. a. becomes upset when reminded of event
   b. becomes upset when in same physical setting in which event occurred
5. when reminded of event, gets anxious, achy, sweaty palms, breathing problems

D: Avoidance

1. a. avoids thinking/talking about event
   b. tries to be unafraid of anything
2. a. avoids activities that remind him/her of event
   b. avoids places that remind him/her of event
   c. avoids people that remind him/her of event
3. can't remember things about event
4. a. has decreased interest in things he/she used to enjoy
   b. has stopped doing things he/she used to enjoy
5. feels cut off from family/friends
6. feels fewer emotions; feels numb
7. a. feels he/she won't grow up
   b. feels he/she will die soon

E: Hyperarousal

1. a. has trouble falling asleep
   b. has trouble staying asleep
2. a. is harder to get along with
   b. is easily angered
3. has difficulty concentrating
4. is super-alert
5. is easily startled, jumpy

Anorexia

1. a. has lost weight by dieting
   b. tries to stay underweight
2. a. current weight and height _____
   b. weight and height when thinnest _____
3. a. is terrified of getting fat
   b. is afraid of gaining weight
   c. fears he/she won't stop eating if he/she starts
4. a. feels fat
   b. feels good/bad depending on weight
   c. thinks his/her weight is a problem
5. if she's started menstruation yet, amenorrhea?

Bulimia

1. eats lots of food in short time
2. feels he/she can't stop eating, only stops because
   _____
3. after eating, tries to lose weight by . . .
   a. not eating
   b. vomiting
   c. taking laxatives
   d. overexercising
4. a. is more weight-conscious than peers
   b. self-image depends on weight

Depression/Dysthymia

A: Dysphoric Mood
1. a. feels sad or depressed
   b. almost every day
   c. lasts most of the day
2. a. feels more irritable
   b. (i) fights (ii) cries (iii) temper
   c. almost every day
   d. lasts most of the day

B: Loss of Interest
1. a. used to have fun doing _____
   b. isn't fun anymore
2. a. wants to have fun but can't
   b. feels that nothing is fun anymore
   c. has lost interest in daily activities

C: Appetite Changes
1. a. has decreased appetite
   b. has lost weight without dieting
   c. clothes are too big now
2. a. has increased appetite
   b. has gained weight

D: Sleep Changes
1. goes to bed @ _____; wakes @ _____
   a. early insomnia
   b. middle insomnia
   c. late insomnia
2. a. naps a lot
   b. hypersomnia

E: Psychomotor Changes
1. a. can't sit still
   b. is fidgety
   c. wrings hands
   d. picks at him-/herself
2. a. takes longer to do things
   b. has difficulty doing anything

F: Low Energy
1. a. has no energy
   b. has to push self
   c. tires easily
   d. sits around, does nothing

G: Guilt
1. a. has bad thoughts about self
   b. feels down on self
   c. feels he/she is no good
   d. hates self
2. a. feels guilty a lot
   b. thinks he/she should be punished

H: Impaired Concentration
1. a. mind has slowed down
   b. forgets things more
   c. has trouble paying attention
   d. listens to teacher less than before
   e. grades have dropped
2. has difficulty making up mind

I: Hopelessness
1. a. feels that nothing good will happen in the future
   b. feels that things won't get any better
   c. feels that there's no hope for the future

J: Morbid/Suicidal Thoughts
1. a. thinks about death
   b. thinks about dead people/pets
2. a. wishes he/she were dead
   b. feels life isn't worth living
   c. has thought of suicide
   d. has thought of suicide plans
   e. has made suicide attempt

Mania/Hypomania

A: Elevated Mood
1. a. feels very, very good
   b. feels wonderful for no reason
   c. is "too high"
2. has discrete periods of irritability

B: Other Symptoms
1. a. believes he/she has special abilities
   b. believes he/she can do things better than anyone
2. a. has lots of energy, no need for sleep
   b. sleeps a lot less without feeling tired
   c. needs ≤3 hours of sleep to feel OK
3. a. has rapid, unstoppable speech
   b. talks so fast that family/friends worry
   c. is told he/she talks too much, too loudly
   d. talks too fast to be understood
4. a. thoughts race through mind
   b. thoughts come too fast to verbalize them all
   c. feels that mind is sped up, working too fast
5. has trouble focusing
6. a. does more things than usual
   b. has more energy than usual
   c. tries many different things
   d. family/friends are concerned
   e. is more active than usual
7. a. gets in trouble more
   b. does things he/she usually wouldn't
   c. gets hurt due to carelessness
   d. is a lot more interested in sex than usual

C: Interference
1. mood/behavior causes problems at (home, school, play)
2. mood/behavior is reason child is here

Enuresis

1. has wet bed after kindergarten
2. a. wets bed at night
   b. wets self during day
3. a. occurs when not sick
   b. is not due to effects of some medication

Encopresis

1. has had bowel movement outside of toilet after kindergarten
2. happens when not sick

Schizophrenia/Psychosis

A: Psychotic Symptoms

1. a. feels someone is out to harm him/her
   b. feels someone is trying to make him/her sick
   c. people seem to be against him/her
   d. people seem to talk about him/her
   e. people spy on him/her
2. a. eyes play tricks on him/her
   b. during daylight
   c. only when falling asleep
   d. ears play tricks on him/her
   e. voices talk about child's feelings/thoughts/acts
   f. voices talk to each other

Interviewer observed:

3. *incoherent speech*
4. *disorganized or catatonic behavior*
5. *inappropriate affect or inability to speak*

B: Interference

1. since problems started, has more difficulty getting along with other people
2. since problems started, does worse in school
3. since problems started, is careless about looks/hygiene

Psychosocial Stressors

A: Child Abuse/Neglect

1. a. M/F criticizes child a lot
   b. M/F wishes child had never been born
   c. M/F says he/she hates child
2. a. M/F ignores child
   b. M/F misses child's doctor appointments
   c. M/F does not feed child
   d. M/F does not clothe child
3. a. child is spanked or hit
   b. child is sometimes spanked or hit for no reason
   c. child fears physical harm from M/F
   d. child has been bruised, sore, taken to doctor
4. child has been sexually abused
5. child has been made to go a whole day without food

B: Other Stressors

1. a. fighting within family
   b. among children
   c. between parents
   d. between parents and children
   e. fighting bothers child
2. child remembers parents' separation/divorce
3. a. family has money problems
   b. child is worried about money problems
4. a. family member is ill
   b. family member has been hospitalized
   c. child worries
5. a. family member drinks or uses drugs a lot
   b. child worries
6. a. family member has been in trouble with police
   b. child worries
7. a. someone close to child has gotten sick and died
   b. child was very upset
8. a. someone close to child was murdered
   b. child was very upset
   c. someone close to child was killed in an accident
   d. child was very upset
9. anything else we need to know so we can help you?
   _____
   _____
10. problems child thinks he/she needs help with?
    _____
    _____
11. anything in the interview that bothered you?
    _____
    _____

P-ChIPS Report Form

Child's Name: _____ Date: _____ / _____ / _____

Informant's Name: _____ Interviewer: _____

Informant's Relationship (circle one): Mother, Father, Stepmother, Stepfather, Guardian, Other _____

Attention-Deficit/Hyperactivity Disorder

A: Inattention
1. a. pays no attention to details
   b. makes careless mistakes on schoolwork
2. can't keep mind on what he/she is doing
3. a. has trouble listening to parent
   b. has trouble listening to teacher
4. has trouble finishing things
5. has trouble organizing self
6. avoids schoolwork
7. loses school supplies
8. a. is easily distracted
   b. teacher reports inattention/daydreaming
9. a. is forgetful
   b. teacher reports forgetfulness

B: Hyperactivity–Impulsivity
1. a. is often told to sit still
   b. is constantly moving hands/feet
2. a. has trouble staying in seat
   b. gets in trouble for getting out of chair
3. gets in trouble for running/climbing
4. a. is too loud when playing
   b. has difficulty playing quietly
5. teacher reports is always "on the go"
6. a. talks out of turn at school
   b. talks too much at home
7. blurts out answers to questions
8. a. pushes ahead in line
   b. can't wait for his/her turn in games
9. a. barges in on other kids' games
   b. pushes into others' groups
   c. interrupts busy people

Oppositional Defiant Disorder
1. a. loses temper when things don't go his/her way
   b. has frequent temper tantrums
2. a. talks back/argues with parents
   b. talks back/argues with teachers
3. a. breaks rules at home
   b. breaks rules at school
   c. refuses to follow teachers' directions
   d. disobeys direct orders
4. purposely "bugs" other people
5. blames others for his/her own mistakes
6. is easily angered by others
7. is angry a lot of the time
8. gets even when angered

Conduct Disorder
1. has stolen >1 time
2. a. lies to get out of doing things
   b. "cons" people
3. has broken into a car or building to steal
4. has skipped school >3 times
5. breaks curfew >1 time per month
6. has run away/stayed out all night >1 time or did not return for a long time
7. a. is a bully
   b. threatens other people
8. a. is avoided because he/she starts fights
   b. gets in trouble for fighting
9. has used a weapon in a fight >1 time
10. a. has hurt someone badly in a fight
    b. has hurt someone for no reason
11. has taken things from people by force
12. has damaged property
13. has set something on fire (>1 time or caused extensive damage)
14. has hurt or killed an animal for fun
15. a. has forcefully performed sexual activity on another
    b. has forced someone to perform sexual activity on him-/herself

Substance Abuse
1. a. has smoked cigarettes ≥2 times _____
   b. has smoked pot ≥2 times _____
   c. has smoked other drugs ≥2 times _____
2. has used alcohol _____
3. has used other drugs _____
4. has sniffed a substance ≥2 times _____

Specific Phobia

1. phobic object/situation: _____
2. when confronted with object/situation,
   a. gets uptight and scared, can't move
   b. cries, clings to parents, throws tantrums
3. a. avoids object/situation
   b. becomes nauseated, feels faint
4. a. fear interferes with (sleep, school, activities)
   b. feels *super* uncomfortable because of fear
5. a. is more scared of object/situation than peers
   b. fear seems silly to child

Social Phobia

1. a. is afraid of being around other people
   b. has fear of performing
2. feels super-uncomfortable when a/b occurs
3. a. tries to avoid social situations
   b. if unavoidable, feels awful
4. a. fear interferes with (sleep, school, activities)
   b. feels *super* uncomfortable because of fear
5. behavior seems silly to child

Separation Anxiety

1. a. cries, begs parent to stay home
   b. tries to stay home with parent at all times
2. a. worries about parent getting harmed
   b. fears parental harm if separated
3. fears personal harm when separated from parent
4. a. has difficulty going to school
   b. refuses to go to school
5. a. is afraid to be in room of house alone
   b. follows parent around the house
6. a. can't sleep if not with parent
   b. can't sleep away from home
7. a. has nightmares about separation
   b. has nightmares about parental loss
8. a. has stomach- or headaches before going to school
   b. gets ill when parent leaves him/her

Generalized Anxiety Disorder

1. worries more than other kids _____
2. a. has difficulty calming down
   b. can't let go of worry
3. when worried, feels edgy, tired, distractible, cranky; has tight muscles, poor sleep

Obsessive-Compulsive Disorder

A: Compulsions

1. does things over and over
2. a. feels behavior will improve things
   b. thinks that if he/she can't perform behavior, something bad will happen
3. feels that behavior does not make sense

B: Obsessions

1. a. has bothersome thoughts/ideas
   b. "sees" pictures in head repeatedly
   c. has to do something but never does it
2. a. tries to make bothersome thoughts go away
   b. tries to pretend that thoughts aren't there
   c. does other things to try to make thoughts go away
3. thoughts seem like child's own (as opposed to someone else putting thoughts in his/her mind)

C: Interference

1. a. thoughts/behaviors cause child discomfort
   b. thoughts/behaviors cause problems at (home, school, play)
   c. thoughts/behaviors interfere with daily routines (time spent daily: _____)

Stress Disorders—PTSD, ASD

A: Exposure

1. a. child experienced traumatic event _____
   b. child witnessed traumatic event happening to someone else _____
2. after event, felt helpless, shocked, horrified, like he/she was falling apart; was hard to calm down
3. how long ago did event happen? _____

B: Dissociation

1. after event, felt cut off from family/friends; felt fewer emotions, felt numb
2. felt out of touch, in a daze
3. felt that the world was not real
4. felt that self was no longer real
5. had trouble remembering event

C: Reexperiencing

1. a. replays event over and over in mind
   b. "sees" event happening again
   c. plays games about event over and over
2. a. has nightmares about event
   b. has nightmares but can't remember what they're about
3. a. "feels" event happening again
   b. acts like event is happening again
4. a. becomes upset when reminded of event
   b. becomes upset when in same physical setting in which event occurred
5. when reminded of event, gets anxious, achy, sweaty palms, breathing problems

D: Avoidance

1. a. avoids thinking/talking about event
   b. tries to be unafraid of anything
2. a. avoids activities that remind him/her of event
   b. avoids places that remind him/her of event
   c. avoids people that remind him/her of event
3. can't remember things about event
4. a. has decreased interest in things he/she used to enjoy
   b. has stopped doing things he/she used to enjoy
5. feels cut off from family/friends
6. feels fewer emotions; feels numb
7. a. feels he/she won't grow up
   b. feels he/she will die soon

E: Hyperarousal

1. a. has trouble falling asleep
   b. has trouble staying asleep
2. a. is harder to get along with
   b. is easily angered
3. has difficulty concentrating
4. is super-alert
5. is easily startled, jumpy

Anorexia

1. a. has lost weight by dieting
   b. tries to stay underweight
2. a. current weight and height _____
   b. weight and height when thinnest _____
3. a. is terrified of getting fat
   b. is afraid of gaining weight
   c. fears he/she won't stop eating if he/she starts
4. a. feels fat
   b. feels good/bad depending on weight
   c. thinks his/her weight is a problem
5. if she's started menstruation yet, amenorrhea?

Bulimia

1. eats lots of food in short time
2. feels he/she can't stop eating, only stops because
   _____
3. after eating, tries to lose weight by . . .
   a. not eating
   b. vomiting
   c. taking laxatives
   d. overexercising
4. a. is more weight-conscious than peers
   b. self-image depends on weight

Depression/Dysthymia

A: Dysphoric Mood

1. a. feels sad or depressed
   b. almost every day
   c. lasts most of the day
2. a. feels more irritable
   b. (i) fights (ii) cries (iii) temper
   c. almost every day
   d. lasts most of the day

B: Loss of Interest

1. a. used to have fun doing _____
   b. isn't fun anymore
2. a. wants to have fun but can't
   b. feels that nothing is fun anymore
   c. has lost interest in daily activities

C: Appetite Changes

1. a. has decreased appetite
   b. has lost weight without dieting
   c. clothes are too big now
2. a. has increased appetite
   b. has gained weight

D: Sleep Changes

1. goes to bed @ _____; wakes @ _____
   a. early insomnia
   b. middle insomnia
   c. late insomnia
2. a. naps a lot
   b. hypersomnia

E: Psychomotor Changes

1. a. can't sit still
   b. is fidgety
   c. wrings hands
   d. picks at him-/herself
2. a. takes longer to do things
   b. has difficulty doing anything

F: Low Energy

1. a. has no energy
   b. has to push self
   c. tires easily
   d. sits around, does nothing

G: Guilt

1. a. has bad thoughts about self
   b. feels down on self
   c. feels he/she is no good
   d. hates self
2. a. feels guilty a lot
   b. thinks he/she should be punished

H: Impaired Concentration

1. a. mind has slowed down
   b. forgets things more
   c. has trouble paying attention
   d. listens to teacher less than before
   e. grades have dropped
2. has difficulty making up mind

I: Hopelessness

1. a. feels that nothing good will happen in the future
   b. feels that things won't get any better
   c. feels that there's no hope for the future

J: Morbid/Suicidal Thoughts

1. a. thinks about death
   b. thinks about dead people/pets
2. a. wishes he/she were dead
   b. feels life isn't worth living
   c. has thought of suicide
   d. has thought of suicide plans
   e. has made suicide attempt

Mania/Hypomania

A: Elevated Mood

1. a. feels very, very good
   b. feels wonderful for no reason
   c. is "too high"
2. has discrete periods of irritability

B: Other Symptoms

1. a. believes he/she has special abilities
   b. believes he/she can do things better than anyone
2. a. has lots of energy, no need for sleep
   b. sleeps a lot less without feeling tired
   c. needs ≤3 hours of sleep to feel OK
3. a. has rapid, unstoppable speech
   b. talks so fast that family/friends worry
   c. is told he/she talks too much, too loudly
   d. talks too fast to be understood
4. a. thoughts race through mind
   b. thoughts come too fast to verbalize them all
   c. feels that mind is sped up, working too fast
5. has trouble focusing
6. a. does more things than usual
   b. has more energy than usual
   c. tries many different things
   d. family/friends are concerned
   e. is more active than usual
7. a. gets in trouble more
   b. does things he/she usually wouldn't
   c. gets hurt due to carelessness
   d. is a lot more interested in sex than usual

C: Interference

1. mood/behavior causes problems at (home, school, play)
2. mood/behavior is reason child is here

Enuresis

1. has wet bed after kindergarten
2. a. wets bed at night
   b. wets self during day
3. a. occurs when not sick
   b. is not due to effects of some medication

Encopresis

1. has had bowel movement outside of toilet after kindergarten
2. happens when not sick

Schizophrenia/Psychosis

A: Psychotic Symptoms

1. a. feels someone is out to harm him/her
   b. feels someone is trying to make him/her sick
   c. people seem to be against him/her
   d. people seem to talk about him/her
   e. people spy on him/her
2. a. eyes play tricks on him/her
   b. during daylight
   c. only when falling asleep
   d. ears play tricks on him/her
   e. voices talk about child's feelings/thoughts/acts
   f. voices talk to each other

Interviewer observed:
3. *incoherent speech*
4. *disorganized or catatonic behavior*
5. *inappropriate affect or inability to speak*

B: Interference

1. since problems started, has more difficulty getting along with other people
2. since problems started, does worse in school
3. since problems started, is careless about looks/ hygiene

Psychosocial Stressors

A: Child Abuse/Neglect

1. a. M/F criticizes child a lot
   b. M/F wishes child had never been born
   c. M/F says he/she hates child
2. a. M/F ignores child
   b. M/F misses child's doctor appointments
   c. M/F does not feed child
   d. M/F does not clothe child
3. a. child is spanked or hit
   b. child is sometimes spanked or hit for no reason
   c. child fears physical harm from M/F
   d. child has been bruised, sore, taken to doctor
4. child has been sexually abused
5. child has been made to go a whole day without food

B: Other Stressors

1. a. fighting within family
   b. among children
   c. between parents
   d. between parents and children
   e. fighting bothers child
2. child remembers parents' separation/divorce
3. a. family has money problems
   b. child is worried about money problems
4. a. family member is ill
   b. family member has been hospitalized
   c. child worries
5. a. family member drinks or uses drugs a lot
   b. child worries
6. a. family member has been in trouble with police
   b. child worries
7. a. someone close to child has gotten sick and died
   b. child was very upset
8. a. someone close to child was murdered
   b. child was very upset
   c. someone close to child was killed in an accident
   d. child was very upset
9. anything else we need to know so we can help you?
   _____
   _____
10. problems child thinks he/she needs help with?
    _____
    _____
11. anything in the interview that bothered you?
    _____
    _____

P-ChIPS Report Form

Child's Name: _____ Date: _____ / _____ / _____

Informant's Name: _____ Interviewer: _____

Informant's Relationship (circle one): Mother, Father, Stepmother, Stepfather, Guardian, Other _____

Attention-Deficit/Hyperactivity Disorder

A: Inattention
1. a. pays no attention to details
   b. makes careless mistakes on schoolwork
2. can't keep mind on what he/she is doing
3. a. has trouble listening to parent
   b. has trouble listening to teacher
4. has trouble finishing things
5. has trouble organizing self
6. avoids schoolwork
7. loses school supplies
8. a. is easily distracted
   b. teacher reports inattention/daydreaming
9. a. is forgetful
   b. teacher reports forgetfulness

B: Hyperactivity–Impulsivity
1. a. is often told to sit still
   b. is constantly moving hands/feet
2. a. has trouble staying in seat
   b. gets in trouble for getting out of chair
3. gets in trouble for running/climbing
4. a. is too loud when playing
   b. has difficulty playing quietly
5. teacher reports is always "on the go"
6. a. talks out of turn at school
   b. talks too much at home
7. blurts out answers to questions
8. a. pushes ahead in line
   b. can't wait for his/her turn in games
9. a. barges in on other kids' games
   b. pushes into others' groups
   c. interrupts busy people

Oppositional Defiant Disorder
1. a. loses temper when things don't go his/her way
   b. has frequent temper tantrums
2. a. talks back/argues with parents
   b. talks back/argues with teachers
3. a. breaks rules at home
   b. breaks rules at school
   c. refuses to follow teachers' directions
   d. disobeys direct orders
4. purposely "bugs" other people
5. blames others for his/her own mistakes
6. is easily angered by others
7. is angry a lot of the time
8. gets even when angered

Conduct Disorder
1. has stolen >1 time
2. a. lies to get out of doing things
   b. "cons" people
3. has broken into a car or building to steal
4. has skipped school >3 times
5. breaks curfew >1 time per month
6. has run away/stayed out all night >1 time *or* did not return for a long time
7. a. is a bully
   b. threatens other people
8. a. is avoided because he/she starts fights
   b. gets in trouble for fighting
9. has used a weapon in a fight >1 time
10. a. has hurt someone badly in a fight
    b. has hurt someone for no reason
11. has taken things from people by force
12. has damaged property
13. has set something on fire (>1 time *or* caused extensive damage)
14. has hurt or killed an animal for fun
15. a. has forcefully performed sexual activity on another
    b. has forced someone to perform sexual activity on him-/herself

Substance Abuse
1. a. has smoked cigarettes ≥2 times _____
   b. has smoked pot ≥2 times _____
   c. has smoked other drugs ≥2 times _____
2. has used alcohol _____
3. has used other drugs _____
4. has sniffed a substance ≥2 times _____

Specific Phobia

1. phobic object/situation: _____
2. when confronted with object/situation,
   a. gets uptight and scared, can't move
   b. cries, clings to parents, throws tantrums
3. a. avoids object/situation
   b. becomes nauseated, feels faint
4. a. fear interferes with (sleep, school, activities)
   b. feels *super* uncomfortable because of fear
5. a. is more scared of object/situation than peers
   b. fear seems silly to child

Social Phobia

1. a. is afraid of being around other people
   b. has fear of performing
2. feels super-uncomfortable when a/b occurs
3. a. tries to avoid social situations
   b. if unavoidable, feels awful
4. a. fear interferes with (sleep, school, activities)
   b. feels *super* uncomfortable because of fear
5. behavior seems silly to child

Separation Anxiety

1. a. cries, begs parent to stay home
   b. tries to stay home with parent at all times
2. a. worries about parent getting harmed
   b. fears parental harm if separated
3. fears personal harm when separated from parent
4. a. has difficulty going to school
   b. refuses to go to school
5. a. is afraid to be in room of house alone
   b. follows parent around the house
6. a. can't sleep if not with parent
   b. can't sleep away from home
7. a. has nightmares about separation
   b. has nightmares about parental loss
8. a. has stomach- or headaches before going to school
   b. gets ill when parent leaves him/her

Generalized Anxiety Disorder

1. worries more than other kids _____
2. a. has difficulty calming down
   b. can't let go of worry
3. when worried, feels edgy, tired, distractible, cranky; has tight muscles, poor sleep

Obsessive-Compulsive Disorder

A: Compulsions

1. does things over and over
2. a. feels behavior will improve things
   b. thinks that if he/she can't perform behavior, something bad will happen
3. feels that behavior does not make sense

B: Obsessions

1. a. has bothersome thoughts/ideas
   b. "sees" pictures in head repeatedly
   c. has to do something but never does it
2. a. tries to make bothersome thoughts go away
   b. tries to pretend that thoughts aren't there
   c. does other things to try to make thoughts go away

3. thoughts seem like child's own (as opposed to someone else putting thoughts in his/her mind)

C: Interference

1. a. thoughts/behaviors cause child discomfort
   b. thoughts/behaviors cause problems at (home, school, play)
   c. thoughts/behaviors interfere with daily routines (time spent daily: _____)

Stress Disorders—PTSD, ASD

A: Exposure

1. a. child experienced traumatic event _____
   b. child witnessed traumatic event happening to someone else _____
2. after event, felt helpless, shocked, horrified, like he/she was falling apart; was hard to calm down
3. how long ago did event happen? _____

B: Dissociation

1. after event, felt cut off from family/friends; felt fewer emotions, felt numb
2. felt out of touch, in a daze
3. felt that the world was not real
4. felt that self was no longer real
5. had trouble remembering event

C: Reexperiencing

1. a. replays event over and over in mind
   b. "sees" event happening again
   c. plays games about event over and over
2. a. has nightmares about event
   b. has nightmares but can't remember what they're about
3. a. "feels" event happening again
   b. acts like event is happening again
4. a. becomes upset when reminded of event
   b. becomes upset when in same physical setting in which event occurred
5. when reminded of event, gets anxious, achy, sweaty palms, breathing problems

D: Avoidance

1. a. avoids thinking/talking about event
   b. tries to be unafraid of anything
2. a. avoids activities that remind him/her of event
   b. avoids places that remind him/her of event
   c. avoids people that remind him/her of event
3. can't remember things about event
4. a. has decreased interest in things he/she used to enjoy
   b. has stopped doing things he/she used to enjoy
5. feels cut off from family/friends
6. feels fewer emotions; feels numb
7. a. feels he/she won't grow up
   b. feels he/she will die soon

E: Hyperarousal

1. a. has trouble falling asleep
   b. has trouble staying asleep
2. a. is harder to get along with
   b. is easily angered
3. has difficulty concentrating
4. is super-alert
5. is easily startled, jumpy

Anorexia

1. a. has lost weight by dieting
   b. tries to stay underweight
2. a. current weight and height _____
   b. weight and height when thinnest _____
3. a. is terrified of getting fat
   b. is afraid of gaining weight
   c. fears he/she won't stop eating if he/she starts
4. a. feels fat
   b. feels good/bad depending on weight
   c. thinks his/her weight is a problem
5. if she's started menstruation yet, amenorrhea?

Bulimia

1. eats lots of food in short time
2. feels he/she can't stop eating, only stops because
   _____
3. after eating, tries to lose weight by . . .
   a. not eating
   b. vomiting
   c. taking laxatives
   d. overexercising
4. a. is more weight-conscious than peers
   b. self-image depends on weight

Depression/Dysthymia

A: Dysphoric Mood
1. a. feels sad or depressed
   b. almost every day
   c. lasts most of the day
2. a. feels more irritable
   b. (i) fights (ii) cries (iii) temper
   c. almost every day
   d. lasts most of the day

B: Loss of Interest
1. a. used to have fun doing _____
   b. isn't fun anymore
2. a. wants to have fun but can't
   b. feels that nothing is fun anymore
   c. has lost interest in daily activities

C: Appetite Changes
1. a. has decreased appetite
   b. has lost weight without dieting
   c. clothes are too big now
2. a. has increased appetite
   b. has gained weight

D: Sleep Changes
1. goes to bed @ _____; wakes @ _____
   a. early insomnia
   b. middle insomnia
   c. late insomnia
2. a. naps a lot
   b. hypersomnia

E: Psychomotor Changes
1. a. can't sit still
   b. is fidgety
   c. wrings hands
   d. picks at him-/herself
2. a. takes longer to do things
   b. has difficulty doing anything

F: Low Energy
1. a. has no energy
   b. has to push self
   c. tires easily
   d. sits around, does nothing

G: Guilt
1. a. has bad thoughts about self
   b. feels down on self
   c. feels he/she is no good
   d. hates self
2. a. feels guilty a lot
   b. thinks he/she should be punished

H: Impaired Concentration
1. a. mind has slowed down
   b. forgets things more
   c. has trouble paying attention
   d. listens to teacher less than before
   e. grades have dropped
2. has difficulty making up mind

I: Hopelessness
1. a. feels that nothing good will happen in the future
   b. feels that things won't get any better
   c. feels that there's no hope for the future

J: Morbid/Suicidal Thoughts
1. a. thinks about death
   b. thinks about dead people/pets
2. a. wishes he/she were dead
   b. feels life isn't worth living
   c. has thought of suicide
   d. has thought of suicide plans
   e. has made suicide attempt

Mania/Hypomania

A: Elevated Mood
1. a. feels very, very good
   b. feels wonderful for no reason
   c. is "too high"
2. has discrete periods of irritability

B: Other Symptoms
1. a. believes he/she has special abilities
   b. believes he/she can do things better than anyone
2. a. has lots of energy, no need for sleep
   b. sleeps a lot less without feeling tired
   c. needs ≤3 hours of sleep to feel OK
3. a. has rapid, unstoppable speech
   b. talks so fast that family/friends worry
   c. is told he/she talks too much, too loudly
   d. talks too fast to be understood
4. a. thoughts race through mind
   b. thoughts come too fast to verbalize them all
   c. feels that mind is sped up, working too fast
5. has trouble focusing
6. a. does more things than usual
   b. has more energy than usual
   c. tries many different things
   d. family/friends are concerned
   e. is more active than usual
7. a. gets in trouble more
   b. does things he/she usually wouldn't
   c. gets hurt due to carelessness
   d. is a lot more interested in sex than usual

C: Interference
1. mood/behavior causes problems at (home, school, play)
2. mood/behavior is reason child is here

Enuresis

1. has wet bed after kindergarten
2. a. wets bed at night
   b. wets self during day
3. a. occurs when not sick
   b. is not due to effects of some medication

Encopresis

1. has had bowel movement outside of toilet after kindergarten
2. happens when not sick

Schizophrenia/Psychosis

A: Psychotic Symptoms

1. a. feels someone is out to harm him/her
   b. feels someone is trying to make him/her sick
   c. people seem to be against him/her
   d. people seem to talk about him/her
   e. people spy on him/her
2. a. eyes play tricks on him/her
   b. during daylight
   c. only when falling asleep
   d. ears play tricks on him/her
   e. voices talk about child's feelings/thoughts/acts
   f. voices talk to each other

> **Interviewer observed:**
> 3. *incoherent speech*
> 4. *disorganized or catatonic behavior*
> 5. *inappropriate affect or inability to speak*

B: Interference

1. since problems started, has more difficulty getting along with other people
2. since problems started, does worse in school
3. since problems started, is careless about looks/hygiene

Psychosocial Stressors

A: Child Abuse/Neglect

1. a. M/F criticizes child a lot
   b. M/F wishes child had never been born
   c. M/F says he/she hates child
2. a. M/F ignores child
   b. M/F misses child's doctor appointments
   c. M/F does not feed child
   d. M/F does not clothe child
3. a. child is spanked or hit
   b. child is sometimes spanked or hit for no reason
   c. child fears physical harm from M/F
   d. child has been bruised, sore, taken to doctor
4. child has been sexually abused
5. child has been made to go a whole day without food

B: Other Stressors

1. a. fighting within family
   b. among children
   c. between parents
   d. between parents and children
   e. fighting bothers child
2. child remembers parents' separation/divorce
3. a. family has money problems
   b. child is worried about money problems
4. a. family member is ill
   b. family member has been hospitalized
   c. child worries
5. a. family member drinks or uses drugs a lot
   b. child worries
6. a. family member has been in trouble with police
   b. child worries
7. a. someone close to child has gotten sick and died
   b. child was very upset
8. a. someone close to child was murdered
   b. child was very upset
   c. someone close to child was killed in an accident
   d. child was very upset
9. anything else we need to know so we can help you?
   _____
   _____
10. problems child thinks he/she needs help with?
    _____
    _____
11. anything in the interview that bothered you?
    _____
    _____

Child's Name: _____ Date: ____ / _____ / _____

Informant's Name: _____ Interviewer: _____

Informant's Relationship (circle one): Mother, Father, Stepmother, Stepfather, Guardian, Other _____

Attention-Deficit/Hyperactivity Disorder

A: Inattention

1. a. pays no attention to details
   b. makes careless mistakes on schoolwork
2. can't keep mind on what he/she is doing
3. a. has trouble listening to parent
   b. has trouble listening to teacher
4. has trouble finishing things
5. has trouble organizing self
6. avoids schoolwork
7. loses school supplies
8. a. is easily distracted
   b. teacher reports inattention/daydreaming
9. a. is forgetful
   b. teacher reports forgetfulness

B: Hyperactivity–Impulsivity

1. a. is often told to sit still
   b. is constantly moving hands/feet
2. a. has trouble staying in seat
   b. gets in trouble for getting out of chair
3. gets in trouble for running/climbing
4. a. is too loud when playing
   b. has difficulty playing quietly
5. teacher reports is always "on the go"
6. a. talks out of turn at school
   b. talks too much at home
7. blurts out answers to questions
8. a. pushes ahead in line
   b. can't wait for his/her turn in games
9. a. barges in on other kids' games
   b. pushes into others' groups
   c. interrupts busy people

Oppositional Defiant Disorder

1. a. loses temper when things don't go his/her way
   b. has frequent temper tantrums
2. a. talks back/argues with parents
   b. talks back/argues with teachers
3. a. breaks rules at home
   b. breaks rules at school
   c. refuses to follow teachers' directions
   d. disobeys direct orders
4. purposely "bugs" other people
5. blames others for his/her own mistakes
6. is easily angered by others
7. is angry a lot of the time
8. gets even when angered

Conduct Disorder

1. has stolen >1 time
2. a. lies to get out of doing things
   b. "cons" people
3. has broken into a car or building to steal
4. has skipped school >3 times
5. breaks curfew >1 time per month
6. has run away/stayed out all night >1 time or did not return for a long time
7. a. is a bully
   b. threatens other people
8. a. is avoided because he/she starts fights
   b. gets in trouble for fighting
9. has used a weapon in a fight >1 time
10. a. has hurt someone badly in a fight
    b. has hurt someone for no reason
11. has taken things from people by force
12. has damaged property
13. has set something on fire (>1 time or caused extensive damage)
14. has hurt or killed an animal for fun
15. a. has forcefully performed sexual activity on another
    b. has forced someone to perform sexual activity on him-/herself

Substance Abuse

1. a. has smoked cigarettes ≥2 times _____
   b. has smoked pot ≥2 times _____
   c. has smoked other drugs ≥2 times _____
2. has used alcohol _____
3. has used other drugs _____
4. has sniffed a substance ≥2 times _____

Specific Phobia

1. phobic object/situation: _____
2. when confronted with object/situation,
   a. gets uptight and scared, can't move
   b. cries, clings to parents, throws tantrums
3. a. avoids object/situation
   b. becomes nauseated, feels faint
4. a. fear interferes with (sleep, school, activities)
   b. feels *super* uncomfortable because of fear
5. a. is more scared of object/situation than peers
   b. fear seems silly to child

Social Phobia

1. a. is afraid of being around other people
   b. has fear of performing
2. feels super-uncomfortable when a/b occurs
3. a. tries to avoid social situations
   b. if unavoidable, feels awful
4. a. fear interferes with (sleep, school, activities)
   b. feels *super* uncomfortable because of fear
5. behavior seems silly to child

Separation Anxiety

1. a. cries, begs parent to stay home
   b. tries to stay home with parent at all times
2. a. worries about parent getting harmed
   b. fears parental harm if separated
3. fears personal harm when separated from parent
4. a. has difficulty going to school
   b. refuses to go to school
5. a. is afraid to be in room of house alone
   b. follows parent around the house
6. a. can't sleep if not with parent
   b. can't sleep away from home
7. a. has nightmares about separation
   b. has nightmares about parental loss
8. a. has stomach- or headaches before going to school
   b. gets ill when parent leaves him/her

Generalized Anxiety Disorder

1. worries more than other kids _____
2. a. has difficulty calming down
   b. can't let go of worry
3. when worried, feels edgy, tired, distractible, cranky; has tight muscles, poor sleep

Obsessive-Compulsive Disorder

A: Compulsions

1. does things over and over
2. a. feels behavior will improve things
   b. thinks that if he/she can't perform behavior, something bad will happen
3. feels that behavior does not make sense

B: Obsessions

1. a. has bothersome thoughts/ideas
   b. "sees" pictures in head repeatedly
   c. has to do something but never does it
2. a. tries to make bothersome thoughts go away
   b. tries to pretend that thoughts aren't there
   c. does other things to try to make thoughts go away

3. thoughts seem like child's own (as opposed to someone else putting thoughts in his/her mind)

C: Interference

1. a. thoughts/behaviors cause child discomfort
   b. thoughts/behaviors cause problems at (home, school, play)
   c. thoughts/behaviors interfere with daily routines (time spent daily: _____)

Stress Disorders—PTSD, ASD

A: Exposure

1. a. child experienced traumatic event _____
   b. child witnessed traumatic event happening to someone else _____
2. after event, felt helpless, shocked, horrified, like he/she was falling apart; was hard to calm down
3. how long ago did event happen? _____

B: Dissociation

1. after event, felt cut off from family/friends; felt fewer emotions, felt numb
2. felt out of touch, in a daze
3. felt that the world was not real
4. felt that self was no longer real
5. had trouble remembering event

C: Reexperiencing

1. a. replays event over and over in mind
   b. "sees" event happening again
   c. plays games about event over and over
2. a. has nightmares about event
   b. has nightmares but can't remember what they're about
3. a. "feels" event happening again
   b. acts like event is happening again
4. a. becomes upset when reminded of event
   b. becomes upset when in same physical setting in which event occurred
5. when reminded of event, gets anxious, achy, sweaty palms, breathing problems

D: Avoidance

1. a. avoids thinking/talking about event
   b. tries to be unafraid of anything
2. a. avoids activities that remind him/her of event
   b. avoids places that remind him/her of event
   c. avoids people that remind him/her of event
3. can't remember things about event
4. a. has decreased interest in things he/she used to enjoy
   b. has stopped doing things he/she used to enjoy
5. feels cut off from family/friends
6. feels fewer emotions; feels numb
7. a. feels he/she won't grow up
   b. feels he/she will die soon

E: Hyperarousal

1. a. has trouble falling asleep
   b. has trouble staying asleep
2. a. is harder to get along with
   b. is easily angered
3. has difficulty concentrating
4. is super-alert
5. is easily startled, jumpy

Anorexia

1. a. has lost weight by dieting
   b. tries to stay underweight
2. a. current weight and height _____
   b. weight and height when thinnest _____
3. a. is terrified of getting fat
   b. is afraid of gaining weight
   c. fears he/she won't stop eating if he/she starts
4. a. feels fat
   b. feels good/bad depending on weight
   c. thinks his/her weight is a problem
5. if she's started menstruation yet, amenorrhea?

Bulimia

1. eats lots of food in short time
2. feels he/she can't stop eating, only stops because
   _____
3. after eating, tries to lose weight by . . .
   a. not eating
   b. vomiting
   c. taking laxatives
   d. overexercising
4. a. is more weight-conscious than peers
   b. self-image depends on weight

Depression/Dysthymia

A: Dysphoric Mood
1. a. feels sad or depressed
   b. almost every day
   c. lasts most of the day
2. a. feels more irritable
   b. (i) fights (ii) cries (iii) temper
   c. almost every day
   d. lasts most of the day

B: Loss of Interest
1. a. used to have fun doing _____
   b. isn't fun anymore
2. a. wants to have fun but can't
   b. feels that nothing is fun anymore
   c. has lost interest in daily activities

C: Appetite Changes
1. a. has decreased appetite
   b. has lost weight without dieting
   c. clothes are too big now
2. a. has increased appetite
   b. has gained weight

D: Sleep Changes
1. goes to bed @ _____; wakes @ _____
   a. early insomnia
   b. middle insomnia
   c. late insomnia
2. a. naps a lot
   b. hypersomnia

E: Psychomotor Changes
1. a. can't sit still
   b. is fidgety
   c. wrings hands
   d. picks at him-/herself
2. a. takes longer to do things
   b. has difficulty doing anything

F: Low Energy
1. a. has no energy
   b. has to push self
   c. tires easily
   d. sits around, does nothing

G: Guilt
1. a. has bad thoughts about self
   b. feels down on self
   c. feels he/she is no good
   d. hates self
2. a. feels guilty a lot
   b. thinks he/she should be punished

H: Impaired Concentration
1. a. mind has slowed down
   b. forgets things more
   c. has trouble paying attention
   d. listens to teacher less than before
   e. grades have dropped
2. has difficulty making up mind

I: Hopelessness
1. a. feels that nothing good will happen in the future
   b. feels that things won't get any better
   c. feels that there's no hope for the future

J: Morbid/Suicidal Thoughts
1. a. thinks about death
   b. thinks about dead people/pets
2. a. wishes he/she were dead
   b. feels life isn't worth living
   c. has thought of suicide
   d. has thought of suicide plans
   e. has made suicide attempt

Mania/Hypomania

A: Elevated Mood
1. a. feels very, very good
   b. feels wonderful for no reason
   c. is "too high"
2. has discrete periods of irritability

B: Other Symptoms
1. a. believes he/she has special abilities
   b. believes he/she can do things better than anyone
2. a. has lots of energy, no need for sleep
   b. sleeps a lot less without feeling tired
   c. needs ≤3 hours of sleep to feel OK
3. a. has rapid, unstoppable speech
   b. talks so fast that family/friends worry
   c. is told he/she talks too much, too loudly
   d. talks too fast to be understood
4. a. thoughts race through mind
   b. thoughts come too fast to verbalize them all
   c. feels that mind is sped up, working too fast
5. has trouble focusing
6. a. does more things than usual
   b. has more energy than usual
   c. tries many different things
   d. family/friends are concerned
   e. is more active than usual
7. a. gets in trouble more
   b. does things he/she usually wouldn't
   c. gets hurt due to carelessness
   d. is a lot more interested in sex than usual

C: Interference
1. mood/behavior causes problems at (home, school, play)
2. mood/behavior is reason child is here

Enuresis

1. has wet bed after kindergarten
2. a. wets bed at night
   b. wets self during day
3. a. occurs when not sick
   b. is not due to effects of some medication

Encopresis

1. has had bowel movement outside of toilet after kindergarten
2. happens when not sick

Schizophrenia/Psychosis

A: Psychotic Symptoms

1. a. feels someone is out to harm him/her
   b. feels someone is trying to make him/her sick
   c. people seem to be against him/her
   d. people seem to talk about him/her
   e. people spy on him/her
2. a. eyes play tricks on him/her
   b. during daylight
   c. only when falling asleep
   d. ears play tricks on him/her
   e. voices talk about child's feelings/thoughts/acts
   f. voices talk to each other

Interviewer observed:
3. *incoherent speech*
4. *disorganized or catatonic behavior*
5. *inappropriate affect or inability to speak*

B: Interference

1. since problems started, has more difficulty getting along with other people
2. since problems started, does worse in school
3. since problems started, is careless about looks/ hygiene

Psychosocial Stressors

A: Child Abuse/Neglect

1. a. M/F criticizes child a lot
   b. M/F wishes child had never been born
   c. M/F says he/she hates child
2. a. M/F ignores child
   b. M/F misses child's doctor appointments
   c. M/F does not feed child
   d. M/F does not clothe child
3. a. child is spanked or hit
   b. child is sometimes spanked or hit for no reason
   c. child fears physical harm from M/F
   d. child has been bruised, sore, taken to doctor
4. child has been sexually abused
5. child has been made to go a whole day without food

B: Other Stressors

1. a. fighting within family
   b. among children
   c. between parents
   d. between parents and children
   e. fighting bothers child
2. child remembers parents' separation/divorce
3. a. family has money problems
   b. child is worried about money problems
4. a. family member is ill
   b. family member has been hospitalized
   c. child worries
5. a. family member drinks or uses drugs a lot
   b. child worries
6. a. family member has been in trouble with police
   b. child worries
7. a. someone close to child has gotten sick and died
   b. child was very upset
8. a. someone close to child was murdered
   b. child was very upset
   c. someone close to child was killed in an accident
   d. child was very upset
9. anything else we need to know so we can help you?
   _____
   _____
10. problems child thinks he/she needs help with?
    _____
    _____
11. anything in the interview that bothered you?
    _____
    _____